Acknowledgments

We would like to thank our friends and clients for their encouragement and help on this project. Our thanks also go to Kirsten Manges, Kristin Jennings, and David Revasch for their professional support.

We would especially like to thank Michael Lavine, who was so generous with his time and took amazing photographs. And Mark Pollard, Kyoko Oshima, and Mako Iijima, who took care of the details. And for their patience and support we owe Dominique Misrahi and Chester Pollard our heartfelt gratitude.

We were fortunate to study Pilates with Romana Kryzanowska, a gifted woman who had the foresight and will to ensure that the work of Joseph Pilates will be preserved and passed on to future generations of instructors. We are proud to call her our teacher.

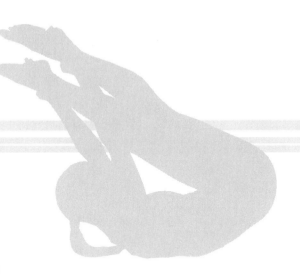

the pilates edge

Karrie **Adamany** and Daniel **Loigerot**

the pilates

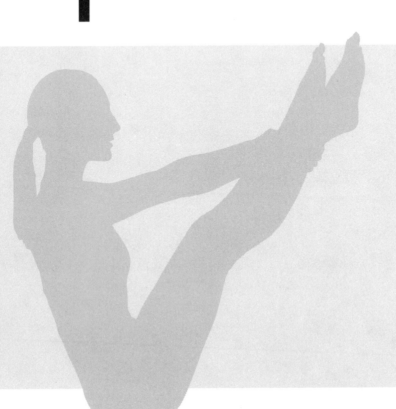

edge

An **Athlete's Guide** to **Strength** and **Performance**

AVERY   a member of Penguin Group (USA) Inc. *New York*

Most Avery books are available at special quantity discounts for bulk purchase for sales promotions, premiums, fund-raising, and educational needs. Special books or book excerpts also can be created to fit specific needs. For details, write Penguin Group (USA) Inc. Special Markets, 375 Hudson Street, New York, NY 10014.

a member of
Penguin Group (USA) Inc.
375 Hudson Street
New York, NY 10014
www.penguin.com

Library of Congress Cataloging-in-Publication Data

Adamany, Karrie.
    The pilates edge : an athlete's guide to strength and
performance / Karrie Adamany and Daniel Loigerot.
        p.   cm.
    Includes index.
    ISBN 1-58333-184-0
        1. Pilates method.   2. Exercise.   3. Physical fitness.
    I. Loigerot, Daniel.   II. Title.
    RA781.A236   2004   2003060022
    613.7'1—dc22

Printed in the United States of America
10   9   8   7   6   5   4   3   2

This book is printed on acid-free paper. ∞

Book design by Mauna Eichner and Lee Fukui

Contents

Foreword

I went to Joseph Pilates as a ballerina with an injured ankle. I was skeptical when he told me that my ankle would heal after only five sessions, but the exercises worked. Ever since, I have been a believer in this method and have dedicated my life to teaching what Joe Pilates taught me.

I have trained many athletes—runners, boxers, skiers, ice skaters, etc.—and the will and determination that these athletes possess goes hand in hand with the basic foundation of Pilates: a focused program based on precision and an overall body awareness is an appropriate method for body preparation and leads to improved performance.

Over the sixty years I have been teaching, I have seen all kinds of people come through the studio doors—healthy, sick, young, old, people who have had serious injuries, and people who have never exercised in their lives, as well as robust athletes. And I have seen people completely transform their bodies and their lives with Pilates.

Utilize this book not only for its intended use—as a tool for athletic preparation—but also as a handbook for healthy living.

—ROMANA KRYZANOWSKA
MASTER TEACHER

Introduction

Most people, regardless of age or ability, consider themselves some-what athletic. Because of this, even the occasional weekend athlete—from someone shooting hoops at the neighborhood park to a family playing their annual Thanksgiving football game—often suffers from some kind of sports-related injury. We have built a system that uses Pilates to improve performance in any sport, as well as to help prevent and rehabilitate injuries. With *The Pilates Edge* you will learn how to approach physical fitness with renewed confidence in your ability to improve your physique and strengthen your game, whatever your sport or level of ability.

It is a seldom-mentioned fact that Joseph Pilates originally trained athletes—boxers (Pilates trained Max Schmeling for his fight against Joe Louis in 1936), gymnasts, circus performers, and later, dancers who worked under both George Balanchine and Martha Graham. Some athletes in recent years who have benefited from Pilates are Martina Navratilova, Chris Evert, Michelle Kwan, Tiger Woods, Annika Sorenstam, NBA player Steve Smith, the Cincinnati Bengals, the San Francisco 49ers, the Oakland Raiders, and members of the New York Giants. The energizing effects a Pilates workout provides makes it ideal for all kinds of athletes in training.

No matter which sport you play, your performance level will improve by practicing Pilates three times per week. Pilates is a safe and effective exercise method that provides the benefits of stretch, strength, and control. It will keep you balanced in the same manner that is necessary for a determined athlete preparing for competition. We cannot attain victory or achieve physical goals without a regular, disciplined practice to make our bodies strong and enduring. This integrated approach to sports training has been proven to work for athletes at all levels.

These routines have been prepared for athletes, but not for athletes alone. They have been designed for the athlete who exists in each of us, for the part of us that wants to overcome physical obstacles and improve ourselves. Anyone can do Pilates, from exercise novices to active people, people with healthy bodies to those with injuries in rehabilitation. We have trained a wide range of people, regardless of their age or body condition, who perform a variety of sports regularly and have seen positive results. So even if you do not consider yourself an athlete, following the Pilates routine in this book will keep you fit and energized for the challenges you face in your daily life.

—Karrie Adamany and Daniel Loigerot

The Essence of Pilates

It may seem obvious that any kind of fitness routine would be benefi-

cial for enhancing performance in sports. But Pilates is superior be-

cause it builds a foundation of strength and flexibility that will create a

better-balanced body. "The Essence of Pilates" is found in the six

principles that make up the foundation on which Pilates is built:

breathing, centering, control, concentration, fluidity, and precision.

All of the principles relate to one another, but taken individually, it is

easy to see how each of the six principles of Pilates plays an important role in training for sports. Using these principles, you will learn total body awareness: you control your mind, your mind controls your body.

A traditional gym workout can get boring after a short time. You find yourself repeating the same training over and over until your mind is wandering, not focusing on the business at hand: improving your body. Pilates re-energizes the mind and body. Regular performance of the routine will lead to increased energy levels and focus as you progress. You will look forward to more physical challenges as you start to feel and see changes in your body. Gradually, as you advance, you will discover the importance of combining all six principles while performing one movement. In the meantime, as you begin, try to simply be aware of how your body is moving. Once the basic principles are understood, it is easy to assimilate more challenging movements at a more rapid pace in order to increase the intensity of the workout.

Principle 1: Breathing

Normally, we breathe without giving it much thought. But breathing creates endurance and energy, while encouraging relaxation. While working through a whole Pilates mat routine, playing a full tennis match, or even nine holes of golf, proper breathing is a vital component to building stamina as it keeps the bloodstream pure by circulating oxygen. While not all Pilates exercises are necessarily "breathing exercises," it is important to be aware of your breathing while exercising. Your breathing will also assist you in performing many of the more challenging movements in the routine.

Principle 2: Centering

The powerhouse—your abdominal muscles, lower back, and buttocks—is your center. Strengthening the abdominal muscles results in a stable pelvis, and a balanced pelvis will support the lumbar spine and keep the feet and legs in alignment. When the body goes out of alignment it cannot perform as efficiently, as your center provides assistance for all movements the body makes. For instance, a runner must keep his core stabilized to gain range and speed. Additionally, a golfer must have a stable center to avoid a lateral shift while swinging the club.

Principle 3: Control

Pilates is best described as a combination of stretch and strength with control. When body and mind operate together, a movement is executed most effectively by using control. All movements in Pilates are initiated from the powerhouse, the center of control. Control is essential in preventing injuries. Without control we always use the same strong muscles and the weaker muscles stay weak. After mastering an exercise, proper control will allow you to do it more quickly, therefore improving your level of performance.

Principle 4: Concentration

Concentration is the focus needed to achieve quality movements. The other five principles become easier to follow once concentration is established. An increased level of concentration enables you to visualize a movement and carry it out to the best of your body's ability. The same principle applies to your golf game: a great deal of focus is required to improve technique. The effectiveness of your Pilates workout or your game will depend on your ability to focus.

Principle 5: Fluidity

Pilates is a complete and graceful choreography in which each exercise leads into the next with energy. Smooth and agile movements create an even, flowing routine that is performed without rushing. It is essential to keep your mind focused on how each movement relates to the next during the workout. Learning to anticipate the next move and carry it out smoothly helps to improve your game and Pilates workout, and will help to conserve energy, an important part of staying in a long game or race, or for a swimmer gliding easily through the water.

Principle 6: Precision

Each movement must be precise due to the fluid nature of the Pilates routine. In Pilates, quality rules over quantity. Fewer precise movements produce the greatest result. More movements than necessary often create fatigue. For example, if a skier does not have efficiency of movement going through the gates he will tire more easily, possibly costing him time. Precision of movement will increase as you become more familiar with the Pilates exercises.

All Pilates exercises are designed to respond to these above-mentioned principles. In addition to using the six principles of Pilates in sports training, you may find that they are applicable to everyday living. Whether bending over to pick up your child, carrying heavy bags, or walking long distances, you will notice great changes in your body, posture, and how you feel when you have incorporated these principles into your daily life.

The Key to Pilates

In addition to the six principles of Pilates, there are a few basic ideas that should be kept in mind in order to make the most of your workout. Below are some of the concepts of Pilates movement that you should become familiar with before beginning your Pilates routine. If this is your first experience with Pilates it is particularly important that you read through the following carefully to gain a better understanding of how your body works while performing the exercises.

POSTURE

When preparing to do Pilates, or any kind of sport, it is first important to establish your posture. Your back, neck, shoulders, hips, and feet should be in proper alignment before you begin. In addition, always be certain that your knees and elbows are not hyperextended, by keeping them straight but not locked.

- Standing posture: An erect yet relaxed standing posture requires that your stomach is lifted, hips and shoulders are square, chest is relaxed, and you are standing with weight equally distributed on both feet.

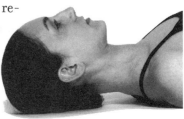

- The neck: Your chin is not lifted, but rather slightly lowered, continuing the long line up from your spine. A long neck also helps to prevent cervical lordosis (forward curvature of the neck) and to relax the jaw muscles. Keep your neck from arching by reaching out through the top of your head.

LONG NECK

- Sitting posture: When sitting in a chair or on the floor be aware of your shoulders and lower back. Lift the stomach in and up so as not to slouch. Lift out of the hips so that your spine is upright, running from the base of the spine to the top of your head.

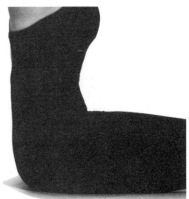

- Shoulder posture: Gravity pulls your shoulders down and forward, creating sloping or slouching. To counterbalance gravity and maintain an upright position, use the opposing muscles in your upper back to pull your shoulder blades down and back, keeping your chest open but not pushed forward.

SITTING POSTURE

Always remember to keep your shoulders relaxed while performing the exercises or your sport, as well as in everyday life. Tension in the shoulders reduces the range of motion and shortens the muscles.

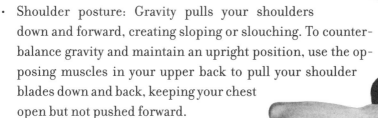

The Powerhouse

SHOULDER POSTURE

Your powerhouse is a band of muscles around your center, which includes your abdominal muscles, lower back, and buttocks. The powerhouse is where all Pilates exercises originate. When properly engaged, it works like a belt around the center of your body, lifting your muscles and lengthening your spine. To engage your powerhouse, stand up tall with shoulders relaxed, "lift" your stomach muscles by pulling them in and up, making sure that you don't allow your ribs to stick out. By doing this, your buttocks will automatically slightly "tuck" under and your spine will lengthen, making you feel taller.

PILATES STANCE

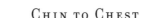

For Pilates stance, make a "V" with your feet, touching your heels together with the toes of each foot about four to five inches apart. Several Pilates exercises are performed with your feet in this position. In Pilates stance, pull your stomach in and up and try to feel your inner thighs opening and the backs of your upper inner thighs squeezing together. Because we are constantly walking in everyday life, in addition to running, biking, etc., the quadriceps do not get adequate rest. Conversely, due to the continual sitting we do daily, the buttocks and inner and outer thighs become soft and lose muscle tone and the hip flexors shorten. A stance with a slight turnout of the legs initiating from the hips will disengage the quadriceps and engage the target area of the buttocks and upper inner and outer thighs.

PILATES STANCE

CHIN TO CHEST

When we say "bring your chin to your chest," it means to gently bring your chin literally to your chest. If you are lying on your back, lift your head slightly so as to look at your stomach. If you are sitting or standing, gently drop your chin to your chest. If you have a weak neck or experience any pain doing this, you may continue the exercise with your head resting down.

CHIN TO CHEST

C-Curve

To find your C-curve, sit on the floor with your knees bent and your feet flat on the ground hip-distance apart. Sit up tall, with your hands gently holding the backs of your thighs. Drop your chin to your chest, looking at your stomach. Make sure to release any tension in your shoulders. From here, draw your stomach in, sinking the abdomen deep into your center, as though you were hollowing it out. Your pelvic bones will tilt up slightly and your shoulders will gently roll in, as your body forms a "C" shape.

Developing your C-curve is an important part of being able to use control while performing the exercises. As your abdominal strength increases, your C-curve will come to you more naturally. Many of the Pilates exercises are performed in this posture, especially the rolling exercises.

The Box

When doing Pilates exercises we always want to perform careful movements within the joint in order to prevent injury. We call this working "in the box." The box is the rectangular outline made if you draw a line from shoulder to shoulder, down to your hip, across to the other hip, and back up to the shoulder. Remember this when doing exercises that require your arms and legs to reach out from your center. Keep your arms in your peripheral vision while doing arm exercises and do not open your legs wider than the width of your mat. By keeping your limbs within the periphery of this box, you avoid the risk of injury and can at the same time focus on precision of movement, a key element in Pilates. When you increase the strength of your muscles by working within the frame of the body, you will be able to exercise more safely.

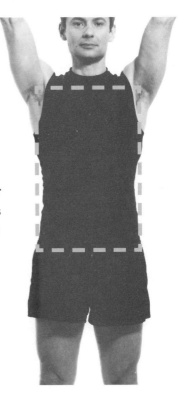

THE BOX

Minimum of Movement

Because Pilates is intended to be a fluid method of exercise, we try to practice minimum of movement between each exercise. This means that there is a seamless transition from one exercise to the next. Once you learn the order of the exercises, practice smooth transitions. This will give you a more complete Pilates workout.

Relaxation

Relaxation plays a big role in doing any form of physical activity, whether it is during an athletic competition or even walking down the street. It is common for people to take stress in their necks, upper, and even lower backs—it is a defensive reaction. When you are performing daily tasks, doing Pilates, or playing sports, release any tension you may be carrying in your shoulders. Remember that the lift and posture you are trying to achieve do not come from raising your shoulders, rather they generate from a strong powerhouse. Release tension in your shoulders by pressing your shoulder blades toward your hips and at the same time try lengthening your spine to the ceiling.

If the body is under stress, you feel tension, which creates discomfort; you unconsciously reduce your range of motion for fear of more pain. Muscle tension also creates spasms that can lead to injury.

Pain and Modifications for Injuries

As with any new physical activity, it is important to consult a physician before beginning. Assuming that you are generally healthy, if you are experiencing any kind of pain or are recovering from an injury, there are modifications that can be made to your Pilates workout:

- For lower back pain: To maintain a flat back when lying down, bend your knees to a 45-degree angle with your feet flat on the mat. If this does not provide enough lower back support, bend your knees to a 90-degree angle with your feet off the mat. This will ensure that there is no strain on your lower back. As your

strength increases and pain decreases, you may want to try to
lift your legs slightly.

· For neck pain: When lying down, keep your head on the mat
instead of bringing your chin to your chest. Once your neck
feels stronger you may want to try to lift your head and gradually incorporate this posture into the appropriate mat exercises. Use a pillow under your neck if you feel a strain on your
neck.

· For knee pain: Keep your knees soft to avoid hyperextension.
Avoid exercises that increase pressure on the knee joint such
as the Squat.

Refer to Chapter 15, Pilates Solutions to Common Sports-Related
Aches and Pains, for more specific explanations of modifications and
injury prevention.

Pilates and Sports

In this chapter you will learn the benefits of incorporating Pilates into your training regimen. You will gain a clear understanding of how you can use the Pilates exercises for your own specific needs in your sports training. You will also learn how to improve your mind/body connection, increase your performance level, and how Pilates can help maintain your health and physical fitness.

Overall Fitness

The Pilates Method allows you to build overall fitness that cannot be achieved with the practice of just one sport. By strengthening the power-house, it develops control from the core, which is central to all movements the body makes. Pilates complements all sports by focusing on breathing, which increases the oxygen supply in the body and builds endurance. You can also use Pilates as a warm-up before practice by loosening the muscles and decreasing stiffness in the joints. It can also help to develop better coordination by sharpening your balance and concentration skills.

Whether you are a professional athlete or a recreational player trying to improve your game and conditioning level, time is always an issue. The Pilates Edge program integrates flexibility and strengthening exercises to help increase your endurance. Few people have the time for an hour of daily stretching, and most people don't save time for the stretch at the end of their workout. With Pilates you stretch while you are doing the exercises, thus saving time to practice your sport. You will gain energy from Pilates that will provide you with the vigor you need to continue your day or practice your sport.

How Pilates Complements Sports Training

- It is an overall fitness builder
- It can correct muscle imbalances due to one-sided training
- It can be used as a restorative process as well as for rehabilitation
- It builds body awareness and focus

Muscle Balance

Some sports develop only a limited range of muscles and many athletes overwork these muscles, which are already strong, neglecting the weaker or smaller muscle groups, which often results in injuries. Adding Pilates as a supplemental training to your regular sport regimen will assure balance in muscle development.

Pilates builds a foundation from the inside out, which means that you build strength in your center (powerhouse) that radiates out to your extremities. You develop muscle groups that are not directly involved in your regular training or sport, which helps to establish stability and muscle balance.

Muscle imbalance can develop especially in sports where one side of the body is dominant, as it is in golf or tennis. Or an imbalance can overload one part of the body as in biking or running, where the lower body is being used more vigorously than the upper body. Because Pilates works the entire body, you can improve your complete physical condition.

Recovery

Constant intensive training and competition tires the body. A process of regeneration is necessary to rebuild energy in addition to preventing injuries. Pilates is a low-intensity aerobic exercise that reverses gravity and releases tension in the joints, which is necessary to restore the body in order to purify the blood and improve blood circulation. An athlete's performance depends on the quick and efficient recovery of stiff, shortened muscles and the capacity to remove the products of fatigue (lactic acid) from the body.

Injury Rehabilitation

It is also important to stay active to facilitate regeneration of tissues (such as cartilage) while rehabilitating injuries. Sitting dormant will only make it more difficult to heal injuries and rebuild muscles. Pilates can get people on their feet more quickly by first strengthening the areas around the injury, then slowly working the injury site itself, providing the movement necessary to get the blood to flow. And since Pilates focuses on proper alignment and attention to range of motion, the Pilates Edge method works with the body, not against it.

Body Awareness

Because all Pilates exercises must be executed with control and concentration, you will become more aware of how your mind controls the body's movements. The six principles of Pilates—breathing, concentration, centering, control, fluidity, and precision—also apply to any sport. Practicing these principles while doing Pilates and sports will build body awareness that can facilitate better performance in your chosen sport.

Pilates can help you locate muscles you don't use during normal, daily activity or in your specific sport. As a result, you will find that your entire body works more efficiently due to better body awareness. You will improve the focus of your workout and your sport through the mind/body connection of Pilates.

The Human Body: Our Musculoskeletal System

In order to comprehend how the body functions in sports, it is first pertinent to review briefly how our muscles work so that we may better understand how to prevent and heal injuries that could otherwise be avoided.

Our skeleton provides the foundation of the body and is held together by muscles, tendons, and ligaments. Muscles are the tissues that contract to produce movement as told by the brain. Fascia separates muscles from adjacent muscles and extends beyond the muscle to form the tendons. Tendons attach the muscle to the bone and have limited elasticity. Ligaments, cartilage, and tendons are called connective tissues. They all help muscles to perform their jobs. The ligaments link bones together at the joints and have no elasticity. Cartilage pads the bones where they meet at the joints.

Muscle tone is important in maintaining correct posture. Muscles that are not used weaken and become atrophied and decrease in size and strength. On the other hand, muscles that are repeatedly used vigorously increase in size and strength and become hypertrophied. If muscles are hypertrophied they may have limited range of motion, whereas atrophied muscles may not be able to maintain stability and mobility function.

The body makes three types of muscle contractions:

- A concentric contraction shortens the muscles and applies force while overcoming resistance (gravity). An example is the Neck Pull (p. 60), where the concentric contraction is in the abdominal muscles on the roll up.

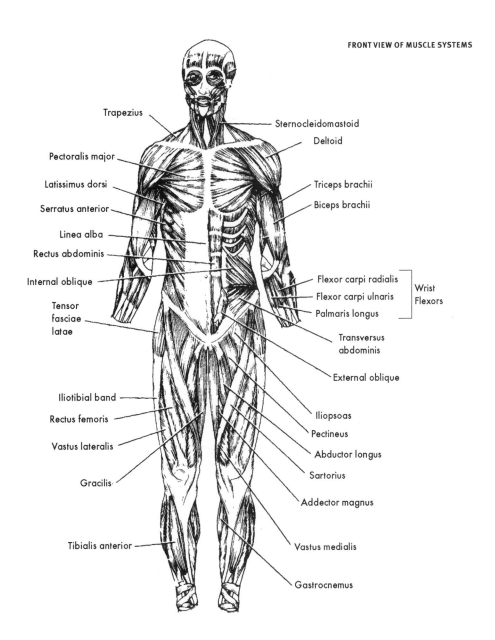

Trapezius

Sternocleidomastoid

Deltoid

Pectoralis major

Latissimus dorsi

Serratus anterior

Linea alba

Rectus abdominis

Internal oblique

Tensor
fasciae
latae

Triceps brachii

Biceps brachii

Flexor carpi radialis

Flexor carpi ulnaris

Palmaris longus

Wrist
Flexors

Transversus
abdominis

External oblique

Iliotibial band

Rectus femoris

Vastus lateralis

Gracilis

Iliopsoas

Pectineus

Abductor longus

Sartorius

Addector magnus

Tibialis anterior

Vastus medialis

Gastrocnemus

- An eccentric contraction occurs when the muscle fibers contract but the whole muscle lengthens, applies force, yet is overcome by resistance (gravity). The Neck Pull can also be used here as the abdominal muscles exert an eccentric contraction on the return to home position.

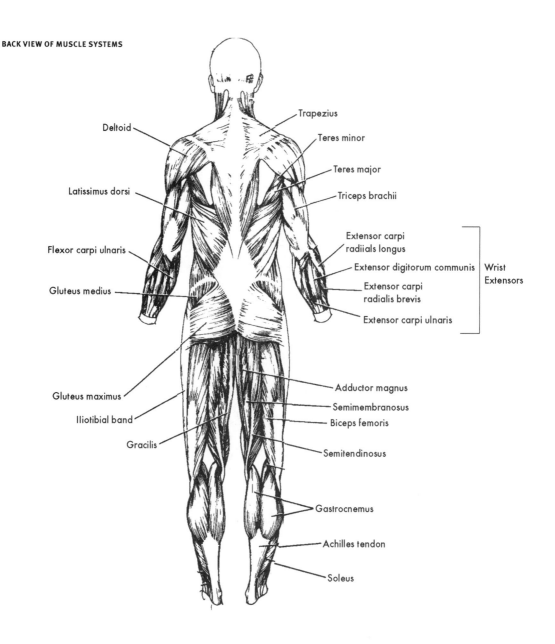

Deltoid

Latissimus dorsi

Flexor carpi ulnaris

Gluteus medius

Gluteus maximus

Iliotibial band

Gracilis

Trapezius

Teres minor

Teres major

Triceps brachii

Extensor carpi radiials longus

Extensor digitorum communis

Extensor carpi radialis brevis

Extensor carpi ulnaris

Wrist Extensors

Adductor magnus

Semimembranosus

Biceps femoris

Semitendinosus

Gastrocnemus

Achilles tendon

Soleus

- An isometric contraction occurs when there is no change to the length of the muscles while applying force—it resists gravity. The Wall Series: Squat (p. 132) engages the leg muscles however the position is held.

Pilates uses all types of muscle contractions in order to develop a balanced body.

The Aerobic and Anaerobic Systems

The energy that the body uses to perform physical activities comes from two sources: aerobic (with oxygen) and anaerobic (without oxygen). The aerobic system produces more energy than anaerobic metabolism without generating lactic acid as a by-product.

Aerobic activities are of longer duration and are constant movements that require the body to receive energy from burning glucose, fatty acids, and amino acids. Anaerobic activities are high intensity and of shorter duration and use glucose as the only fuel to produce energy. The glycogen, the storage form of glucose, can be found in the muscles and liver cells.

The body's heart rate is lower during aerobic exercise than during anaerobic exercise. Thus aerobic training works your heart and lungs and improves total physical fitness. Pilates, due to its steady, fluid nature, is a low-impact aerobic workout because it uses breathing to increase endurance. Therefore Pilates increases the body's capacity to perform better in sports and maintain a constant condition. Aerobic exercise also burns fat, which means weight loss is an additional benefit of Pilates.

Anaerobic energy production is anaerobic glycolysis (glycolysis involves breaking down the carbohydrates from your diet into glucose). A by-product of anaerobic glycolysis is lactic acid. With continued high-intensity muscle work, lactic acid accumulates in the muscles and is responsible for the burning sensation. By training, the body becomes better at quickly removing the lactic acid from the working muscles during recovery. Athletes with better aerobic fitness levels can clear the accumulated lactic acid from the working muscles more rapidly than individuals with less aerobic fitness. When you get a cramp in your muscles, it means that your muscle is locked in a painful and sustained spasm. The cause is often exercise-induced dehydration. Immediate relief can be obtained by a gentle stretch and by drinking fluids. Cramps are usually minimal for Pilates practitioners

You can measure exercise intensity by taking your pulse. To take your pulse, place two fingers approximately one inch below your left wrist joint or two fingers at the side of your neck just below the jawbone. Take your pulse for 10 seconds then multiply that number by 6 for the minute-long value. If you don't want to stop your workout to take your pulse you can use the rate of perceived exertion: if you are able to hold a conversation while exercising you are still in the optimal training zone. If not, you are in the anaerobic zone.

You can then estimate your maximal heart rate by using the following equation:

Maximal heart rate (MHR) = 220 − your age.

To work your heart and lungs most efficiently and burn fat you need to aim to work at between 65 and 85 percent of your maximum heart rate, which is your optimum training zone. For example, for a 40-year-old person:

$$220 - 40 = 180$$
$$180 \times .65 = 117$$
$$180 \times .85 = 153$$

This person should aim at keeping their heart rate above 117 but below 153.

as stretching is part of many of the exercises.

Pilates energizes your body and increases its endurance by improving your circulation and breathing by creating a greater exchange of oxygen between the blood and working muscles. Proper breathing is central to every Pilates exercise. When you exercise, your heart rate increases, which boosts circulation and drives fresh blood to the capillaries. If you exercise regularly the long-term benefits can be reduced blood pressure and lower risk of heart attack.

Pilates does not only provide physical benefits. When exercising your body releases adrenaline as well as serotonin, a chemical that makes you feel happy. Together with increased levels of oxygen in the blood, these produce the general sense of well-being that follows a Pilates workout. So regular workout sessions can help to release tension and decrease stress, which is a very important task in our fast-paced lifestyles.

We have created the specific Pilates sport routines in this book based on the individual needs of the athletes, according to their goals and common demands on the body in their sport. Each exercise in a given routine addresses the demands of that particular sport. The efficiency of movement in Pilates translates to sports: one must not expend more energy than necessary to get the job done.

In order to get the most out of your sport workout, it is first important to work through the traditional Pilates mat program. Jumping into one exercise doesn't work—you need to first build a good foundation.

Pilates can become a part of your lifestyle in which you can achieve peak conditioning and a healthy body.

Of course regular practice is necessary to get the desired results. You will see in each individual sport chapter two different routines—(1) intermediate/ advanced and (2) more advanced—and the number of times per week they should be practiced. We are confident that with commitment to the Pilates Edge Program you will see your desired results.

PERCENTAGE OF MAXIMUM HEART RATE		
AGE	**65%**	**85%**
18–25	130	169
26–30	127	163
31–36	124	158
37–42	120	153
43–50	116	147
51–58	112	141
59–65	108	134
65+	104	129

3

The Pilates Program

The Pilates routine is performed in a specific order for a very basic yet important reason: Pilates is based on the premise that the body requires strengthening and stretching, and that opposing movements are needed in order to build a balanced body. To that end, follow the routine carefully, but remember to omit any exercises that cause you any pain or discomfort. Be methodical about your workout, working slowly at first to make sure you are doing the exercises properly. Refer to Chapter 1 to review the Key to Pilates whenever necessary.

On the following pages you will find the Pilates exercises with these components:

Level The level of the exercise, either Beginner, Intermediate, or Advanced.

Emphasis The emphasis listed in parentheses is the goal you should keep in mind while performing the exercise, which will either be strength, control, and/or mobility.

Tip Advice on how to better perform the exercise.

Modification If you are unable to perform the exercise as it is given, we offer modifications to make it easier. If there is no modification listed, and especially if you have an injury, omit the exercise until you have enough strength to properly execute the movement.

Advanced Challenge When you master the given exercise, we have in some cases included an additional challenge to the movement.

Benefit for Sports How the exercise relates to sports and can help you perform better.

Transition How to go from one exercise to the next.

Repetition One complete movement of a particular exercise.

Set A group of repetitions performed in sequence.

A standard exercise mat should be used for Pilates floor exercises, or a towel can substitute for a mat when you are traveling. It is important to have enough space around you in order to rotate your arms and legs in a circle while standing, sitting or lying down. It is sometimes helpful to have a mirror to check your position, but it is not necessary. You may rest between exercises, but keep in mind that the ultimate goal is to seamlessly transition from one movement to the next. A workout, at the beginner or advanced level, should take you between 20 and 30 minutes. Unless specifically noted, **breathe** normally.

A commitment to a regular Pilates practice will result in the desired effect—be it a better time, injury prevention or overall fitness. Enjoy your workout!

The Hundred (Strength)

- Begin by lying flat on the mat with your arms straight at your sides. Bend your knees into your chest at a 90-degree angle.

- Lift your arms 4 to 6 inches from the mat. Create a pumping motion by lowering your arms until the palms are just above the ground and then raising them to the starting position. Keep your arms straight throughout the movement.

- Take one deep inhalation through the nose for 5 counts, then one full exhalation through the mouth for 5 counts. One count should coincide with one arm pump.

- Once you have mastered the breathing, lift your head, bringing your chin to your chest.

- Straighten your knees so that your legs are perpendicular to your body, forming a 90-degree angle, and continue pumping and breathing.

- Repeat 10 sets of 5 reps breathing in and 5 reps breathing out.

Tip: Draw your stomach into your spine. Use the energy of the arms and hips reaching in opposition to take pressure out of the quadriceps muscles (thighs).

Modification: For lower back pain, keep legs slightly bent or legs bent at a 90-degree angle. For neck pain, keep head on mat or use cushion.

Advanced Challenge: As your abdominal muscles grow stronger, try to lower your legs as you keep them straight. You may also add more repetitions up to 200.

Benefit for Sports: Build endurance; strengthen torso; stabilize spine, which is good for serve/swing control in tennis/golf, and prevent back injury.

Transition: Bend knees into your chest. Then lie flat on your back with your legs straight on the ground for the Roll Up.

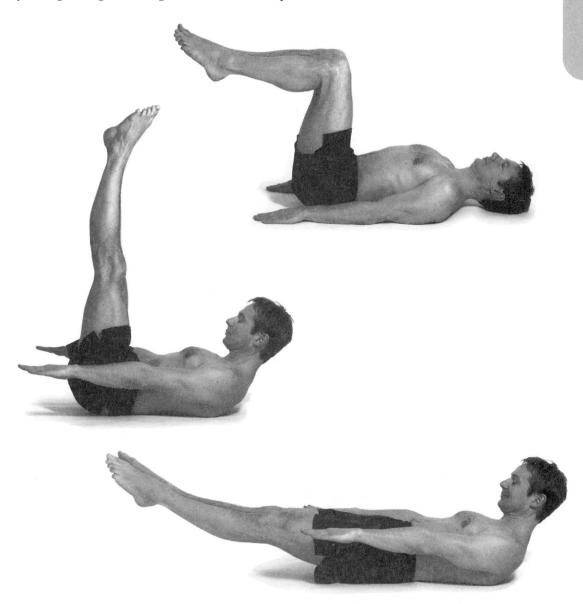

Roll Up (Strength/Mobility)

- Lie on your back with your legs straight and your feet in Pilates stance.

- Lift your arms by your ears, shoulder distance apart.

- Lift your head and bring your chin to your chest. Inhale. Lift your arms to the ceiling and start to roll up to sitting. Draw your stomach in deep, reaching your arms forward.

- Exhale as you reach beyond your toes, keeping your stomach from touching your thighs. Your arms should remain shoulder height.

- Inhale, draw your stomach in, and begin to roll back down, keeping in mind your C-curve. Exhale as you complete the movement by touching each vertebra consecutively on the mat until you are lying flat again with arms by your ears.

- Repeat 3 to 5 times.

Tip: Draw the stomach in deeper when rolling up so as not to use your arms to pull you up. This is a slow, controlled movement.

Modification: Slightly bend your knees with feet on the floor, and keep your arms by your side if you cannot roll up smoothly.

Benefit for Sports: Back injury prevention; swing/serve control in golf and tennis; and flexibility.

Transition: Lie flat on the mat. Intermediate go to Single Leg Circles, Advanced go to Roll Over.

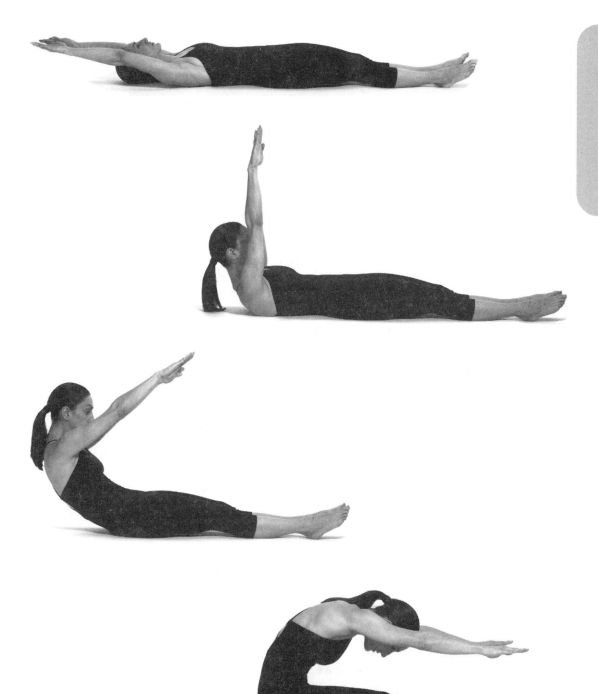

Roll Over (Control)

- Lie flat on the mat with your arms at your side. Bring your legs together in Pilates stance. Pointing your toes, bring your legs up straight until they are perpendicular with your body, concentrating on using your powerhouse.

- Inhale and lift your buttocks up and off the mat, bringing the legs straight overhead and parallel to the floor, with your toes touching the floor above your head.

- Exhale. Open your legs to shoulder width, and flex your feet as you start to slowly roll down your spine, keeping your legs close to your chest.

- When your tailbone reaches the mat and your legs are up at a 90-degree angle, close your legs, point the toes, and repeat the exercise 2 more times.

- Then reverse the position of your feet, i.e., legs open and toes pointed to roll over, closed and flexed to roll down.

- Perform 3 times on each side.

Tip: Initiate the movement with the powerhouse (not the legs) when rolling over.

Modification: Begin and end with legs straight at a 90-degree angle if you cannot keep your back flat when lowering your feet to the floor.

Advanced Challenge: When your tailbone reaches the mat, continue to lower your legs as close as possible to the mat while maintaining your entire spine on the mat.

Benefit for Sports: Prevent lower back pain; torso stability and flexibility.

advanced

Transition: Bring one leg down and keep one leg straight up at 90 degrees for Single Leg Circles.

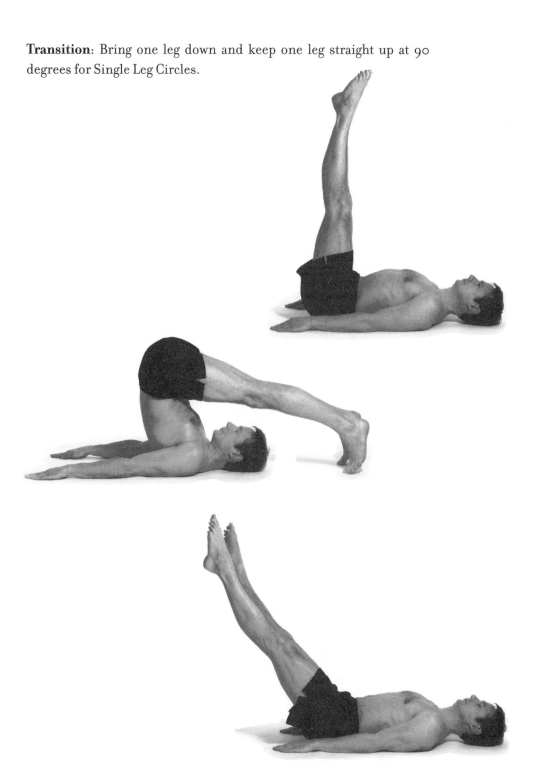

Single Leg Circles (Mobility)

- Lie flat on your back with your arms by your sides.

- Reach one leg up to the ceiling, while the other leg reaches straight down the center line of your body on the mat.

- Slightly rotate the leg, reaching for the ceiling out from the hip. Begin to make circles, first crossing your body with your leg.

- Start and stop the circle at your nose—the center of your body— and work within the frame of your body (the box).

- Repeat 5 times, then reverse the circles 5 times.

Tip: Initiate the movement from your hip and keep your leg loose. The energy of the circle is on the way up.

Modification: If you feel a strain in the back of your knee, keep it slightly bent.

Advanced Challenge: You can make bigger circles as long as the hips are steady.

Benefit for Sports: Regenerate tired legs; prevent hamstring injury for runners and cyclists.

Transition: Bring both legs down to the mat then sit up for Rolling Like a Ball.

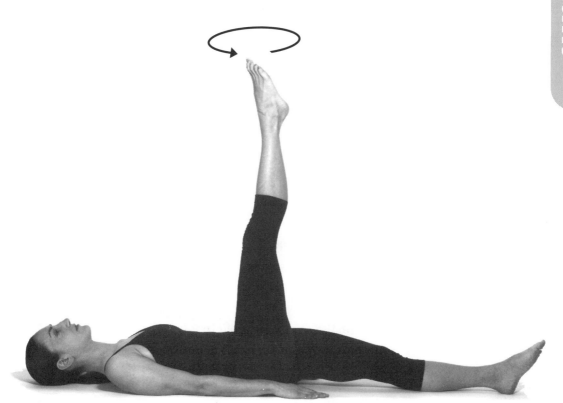

Rolling Like a Ball (Control)

- From a seated position, bring your knees close to your chest. Holding on to your ankles, bring your head down to your knees. Stay in a tight ball by keeping your feet close to your buttocks and the stomach pulled in.

- Inhale. Roll back to your shoulders and exhale. Roll back up to sitting, holding the position on the up. Balance on your sitting bones for 2 counts.

- Repeat 6 times.

Tip: Keep your head close to or between your knees.

Modification: If you have knee pain, try it with your knees bent, holding on to the backs of your thighs.

Advanced Challenge: Place your right hand on the left ankle and the left hand on the right wrist. Hold your feet close to your buttocks.

Benefit for Sports: Improve balance, control; stabilize torso, especially for cycling and skiing; prevent back injury; and release body tension.

Transition: In a sitting position, place your right hand on your right ankle and your left hand on your right knee. Then lower your torso down to the mat while keeping your knee close to your chest for the Single Leg Stretch.

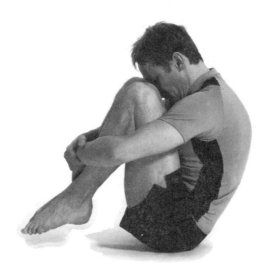

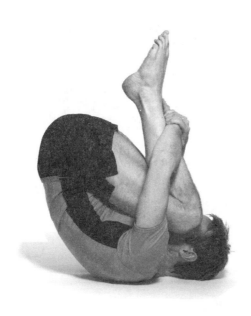

Single Leg Stretch (Strength)

- Lying flat on the floor, bring your head up and your chin to your chest. Bend your right leg into your chest, placing your right hand on your right ankle, and your left hand on your right knee.

- Lift the left leg a few inches off the mat.

- Switch legs, pulling your left knee into your chest and stretching your right leg straight in front of you, keeping it off the mat.

- Repeat 10 times for 5 sets.

Tip: Keep the box (hip and shoulders) square, with a flat back and hips, knees, and feet in alignment.

Modification: For knee pain, place your hands under your knees. For back pain, bring your legs higher.

Advanced Challenge: Try to touch the mat with your toes when extending the leg for deeper abdominal work.

Benefit for Sports: Stabilize torso; thigh and hamstring flexibility; and prevent back injury.

Transition: Bring both knees into your chest to prepare for the Double Leg Stretch.

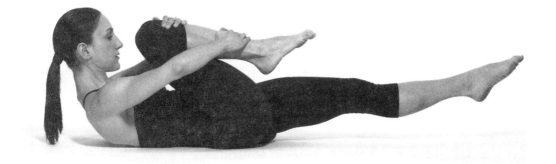

Double Leg Stretch (Strength)

- Lying flat on the mat, bring both knees into your chest, holding on to your ankles.

- Inhale. Extend both arms and legs straight out at opposite 45-degree angles.

- Stretch your arms out to the side, making a circle, and exhale. Reach for your ankles as you pull your knees back into your chest.

- Repeat 5 to 10 times.

Tip: Draw your stomach in to your spine. Try to stretch your sitting bones away from your powerhouse to lengthen your entire body. Keep your feet above your hip bones to avoid arching your back.

Modification: For knee pain, place your hands under your knees. For back pain, keep your legs higher. For shoulder pain, do not make circles with the arms, simply raise and lower them down to grab your ankles.

Advanced Challenge: When beginning the leg extension, touch the toes to the mat while legs are still bent for deeper abdominal work.

Benefit for Sports: Prevent lower back pain; stabilize torso; improve flexibility for swimming; improve breathing for swimming, skiing, running, and cycling.

Transition: Beginner go to Spine Stretch Forward. Intermediate, raise right leg straight up in the air and hold on to your ankle with both hands to prepare for Single Straight Leg.

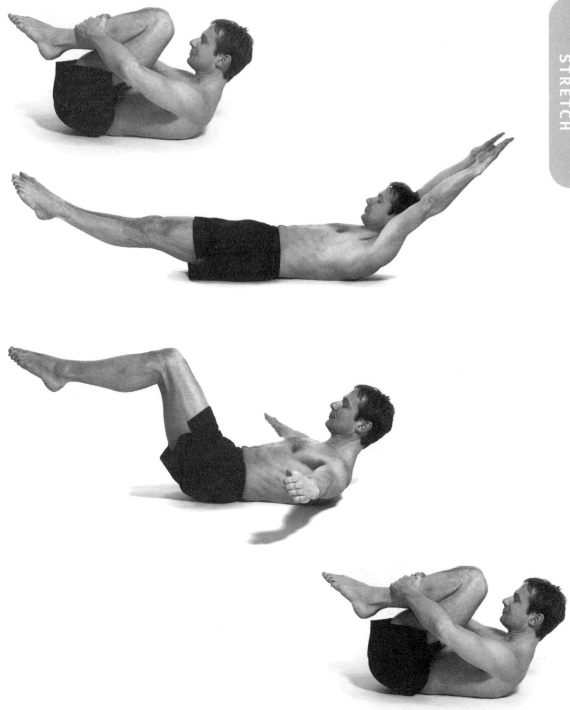

Single Straight Leg (Strength/Mobility)

- Lying on your back with your knees bent to your chest, bring your head up and your chin to your chest. Lift your right leg and grab your ankle with both hands.

- Pull the leg to you, keeping it straight, as you extend your left leg straight out a few inches above the mat.

- Scissor your legs through the air, pulling the left leg to you, grasping it at the ankle, and stretching the right leg out a few inches above the mat.

- Alternate legs 10 times.

Tip: Inhale/exhale every other rep. Bring your leg to your hands and not the opposite.

Modification: For back pain, keep the extended leg higher. For bad knees, place your hands behind your knees instead of ankles.

Advanced Challenge: Instead of grasping your ankles, keep your arms straight alongside your body two inches off the mat as you scissor the legs.

Benefit for Sports: Stabilize the torso; hamstring flexibility.

Transition: Lift both legs straight up at a 90-degree angle for the Double Straight Leg.

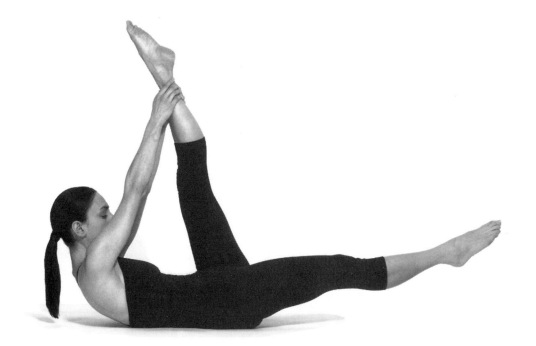

Double Straight Leg (Strength)

- Lying on your back with your legs straight, bring your head up and your chin to your chest with your hands behind your head and your elbows reaching out to the sides.

- Raise your legs straight to a 90-degree angle, keeping them in Pilates stance.

- Draw your stomach in and up, inhale, and lower your legs together. Go as low as you can go while keeping your back flat on the mat.

- Exhale and bring your legs back up.

- Repeat 5 to 10 times.

Tip: Remember that you must keep your lower back on the mat and stabilize your pelvis with the powerhouse.

Modification: For back pain, only lower the legs as low as they can comfortably go and/or place your hands under your buttocks.

Advanced Challenge: Try to touch the mat with your heels when lowering your legs.

Benefit for Sports: Prevent back injury; control.

Transition: Bend both knees into your chest for the Criss Cross.

intermediate

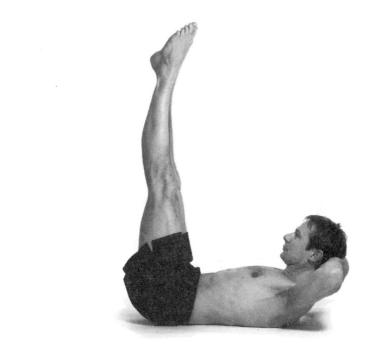

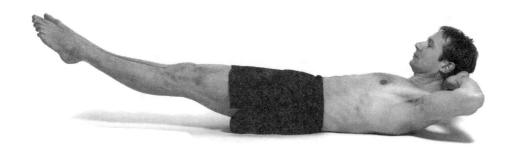

Criss Cross (Strength)

- Lying on your back with your legs straight, bring your head up and your chin to your chest with your hands behind your head and elbows reaching out to the sides.

- Slightly lift your upper body until your shoulders are off the mat. Inhale. Bend your right knee up to your chest and bring your left elbow to meet your knee. Keep your left leg extended straight to 45 degrees.

- Turn your head as you rotate your shoulders to the right and look at your right elbow. Keep both elbows open wide. Hold for 3 counts, exhale, and come to center.

- Inhale again as you switch sides.

- Repeat 3 sets.

Tip: Work within the frame of the body, being careful not to shift to one side. Only the upper body twists.

Advanced Challenge: Keep your knee bent at a 90-degree angle and bring your elbow up to meet the knee.

Benefit for Sports: Improve spinal rotation; torso strength for golf, tennis, and skiing.

Transition: Bend your knees into your chest and place your head on the mat (Spine Release Position) to relax. Sit up for the Spine Stretch Forward.

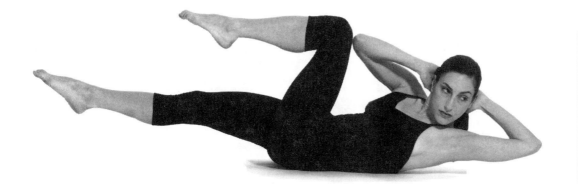

Spine Stretch Forward (Mobility)

- Sit up tall with your legs straight at the outer edges of the mat and your feet flexed. Extend your arms in front of you, shoulder-height and shoulder-width apart.

- Inhale as you squeeze your buttocks, lift your pelvic floor muscles, and sit up taller. Reach forward, bringing your chin to your chest and rolling down your spine.

- Your stomach should continue lifting, as though you are coming up and over a big ball. Keep reaching your arms in front of you, with your shoulders relaxed. Exhale.

- Inhale as you start to roll back up using your powerhouse. Reach your fingers forward as you continue to lift up to sitting tall.

- Keep lifting through your stomach when you reach the top. Exhale.

- Repeat 3 to 5 times.

Tip: Keep in mind that it is a stretch for the spine and not only for the backs of thighs. Also remember to keep your quadriceps relaxed.

Modification: For back or knee pain, slightly bend the knees. Or you may sit on a cushion to have your hips slightly higher than your feet.

Advanced Challenge: For an extra stretch through the legs, grab your toes, but remember to always keep your stomach lifted. Bring the top of your head to the mat to increase the curve of the spine.

Benefit for Sports: Back and hip injury prevention.

Transition: Bend your knees and draw your feet in close to your body by grasping the tops of your ankles.

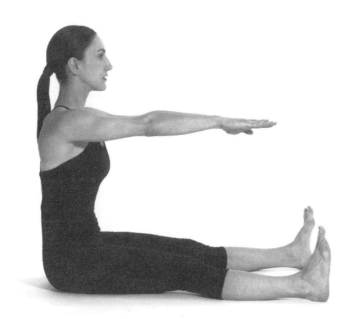

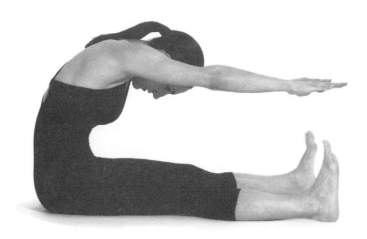

Open Leg Rocker (Control)

- Sitting up tall, bend your knees and grasp the tops of your ankles to draw your feet close to your body.

- Straighten your legs out so your body is in a "V" position with your legs about shoulder-width apart. You should be balancing on your sitting bones.

- Inhale. Engage your powerhouse and bring your chin to your chest. Keeping your body in the "V" position, roll your body back, taking your legs overhead, being careful not to roll onto your neck.

- Using your powerhouse—not momentum—roll back up and balance at the top in the "V" position. Exhale.

- Repeat 6 times.

Tip: Make sure to draw in from the abdomen before rolling back and up. Try not to pull your legs with your arms when rolling up.

Modification: For neck pain, simply hold the balance with your legs extended and do not roll back.

Advanced Challenge: Bring your feet together and grab your ankles (or toes) and do the Closed Leg Rocker.

Benefit for Sports: Balance; control.

Transition: Keep your legs elevated and bring them straight together in front of you. Slowly roll your upper body down to the mat, keeping your legs up straight at a 90-degree angle for the Corkscrew.

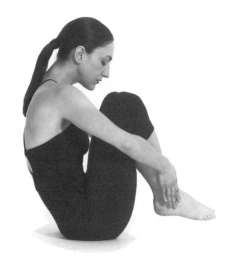

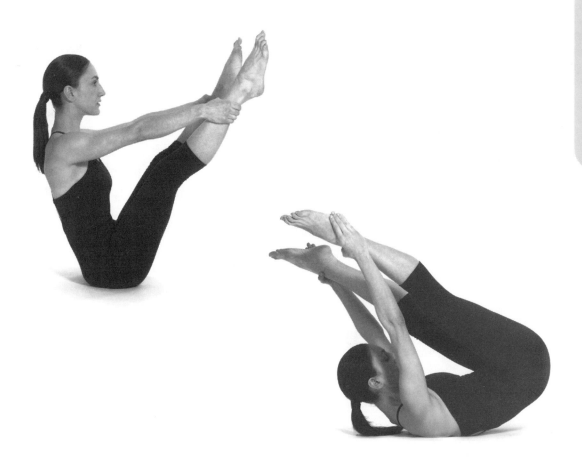

Corkscrew (Control/Strength)

- Lie flat on the mat with your legs straight, making a 90-degree angle with your body. Your arms are straight down by your sides.

- With your feet in Pilates stance, make a small circle with your legs beginning on the right, circling down and around to the left, and back up to center.

- Reverse the direction of the circle, beginning on the left side.

- Repeat 3 times each, alternating the direction.

Tip: Keep your hips anchored into the mat while the legs are rotating, controlling the movement with your powerhouse.

Modification: For back pain, place your hands under your buttocks and reduce the range of motion.

Advanced Challenge: As you feel stronger, try to start lifting the first four vertebrae off the mat as your legs return to center. For a greater challenge, begin the exercise with the legs lifted straight to the ceiling, lower back lifted off the mat and weight on your shoulders. To make the circles, first slightly twist your hips in the air before angling down onto one hip, circling down around, and coming back up on the other hip, and pushing the legs straight up to the ceiling.

Benefit for Sports: Trunk stability; increase range of motion in hips for skiing.

Transition: Sit up for the Saw.

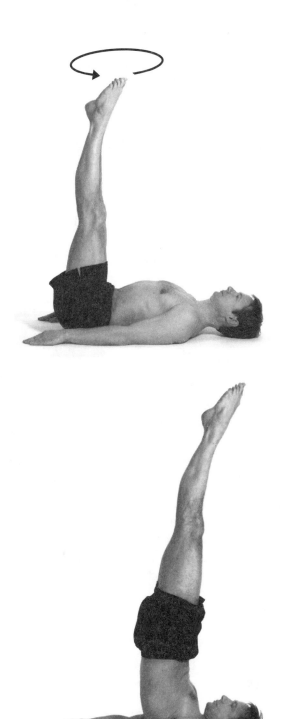

ſaw (Mobility)

- Sit up tall with your legs extended out at the side edges of the mat. Stretch your arms out to your sides at shoulder height.

- Inhale as you lift from your center, squeezing your buttocks and pressing your sitting bones into the mat. Twist the spine to the right, reaching your left hand down to the outside of your right foot. The right arm reaches back as you stretch in both directions, without bouncing.

- Exhale the air out of your lungs completely, keeping the stomach lifted, feeling the opposing stretch with your arms.

- Inhale as you roll back up to center and twist to the other side and exhale.

- Repeat 3 times.

Tip: Keep your hips square and anchored into the mat—this is a stretch for the waist/spine rather than your arms.

Modification: For severe stiffness in the legs or back, slightly bend the knees. Or sit on a cushion so that your hips are slightly higher than your feet.

Benefit for Sports: Torso rotation for tennis, golf, swimming, and skiing; back injury prevention.

Transition: Bring your legs together and turn onto your stomach for the Neck Roll.

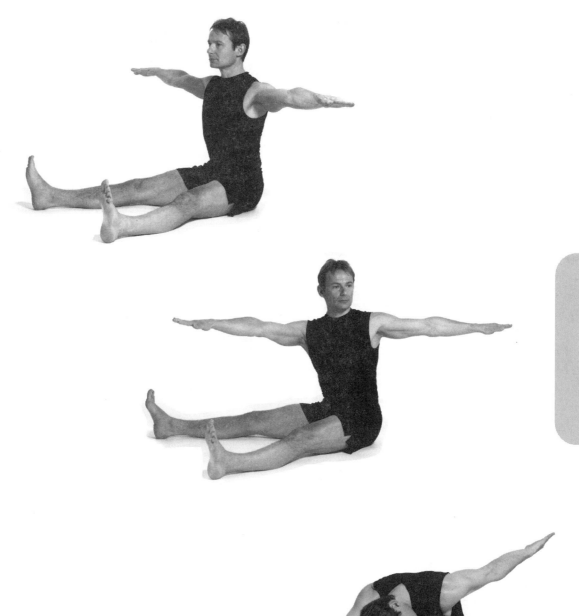

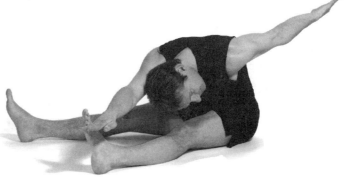

Neck Roll (Mobility)

- Lie on your stomach with your legs together and your face down on the mat. Bend your arms close to the body and place your hands just under your shoulders. Your elbows should be pointing backward.

- Engage the powerhouse. Pressing into the mat with your hands and forearms, push your upper body up. Keeping your shoulders down and your neck long, straighten your arms as much as you feel comfortable.

- Turn and look to one side, roll your neck to look down, then up to the other side. Reverse. Do this slowly.

- Repeat, rolling the neck in the opposite direction.

Tip: Make sure to lift abdominal muscles to support your lower back.

Modification: For back pain, begin the exercise with your forearms into the mat.

Benefit for Sports: Cervical spine mobility for golf, cycling, swimming, and tennis; invert the spine and spinal stability.

Transition: Intermediate go to Single Leg Kick, Advanced go to Swan.

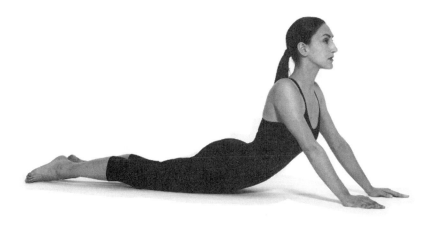

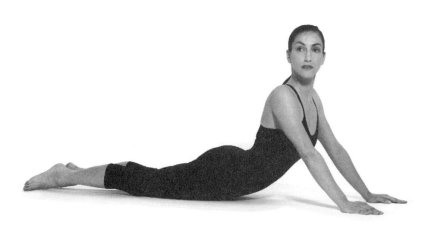

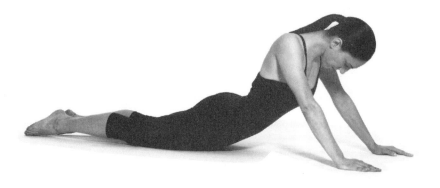

ʃwan (Mobility/Strength)

- Lie on your stomach with legs together and elbows bent backward with palms flat on the mat. Lift your chest and upper body off the mat and squeeze the inner thighs together.

- Engage abdominal muscles and exhale. Rock forward on your stomach and reach your arms in front of you with palms up as you lift your legs. Your arms should be by your ears with your hands pointing over your head.

- Inhale as you rock in the reverse direction, lowering your feet and lifting your arms and chest. Your arms should still be pointed over your head close to your ears.

- Repeat 6 times.

Tip: Keep your abdominal muscles engaged to support your spine. Keep your legs together, engaging your thighs and buttocks. The whole body must stay lifted while doing this exercise—do not use just your arms to create the movement.

Benefit for Sports: Invert the spine to prevent kyphosis (accentuated curvature of the thoracic spine).

Transition: Sit back on your heels to open your lower back (Spine Stretch Release, p. 285). Return to your stomach for Single Leg Kick.

advanced

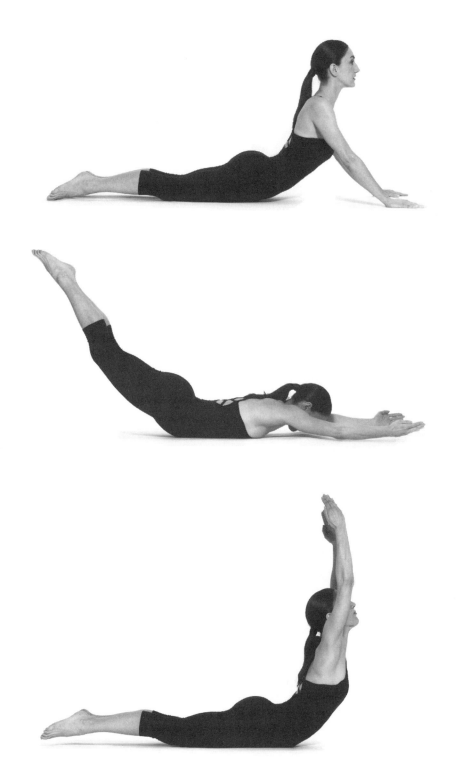

Single Leg Kick (Strength)

intermediate

- Lie on your stomach and prop up your torso by resting on your forearms with your fists together in front of your chest. Your elbows should be pointed out to the side so that your arms make a diamond shape.

- Push your fists together and lift your abdominal muscles, chest, and head.

- With your right leg, kick your buttocks 2 times, then alternate and use your left leg. Exhale as you kick and inhale as you lower the leg.

- Repeat 5 times with each leg.

Tip: Keep lifting the powerhouse while kicking, keep your legs together, and kick with energy.

Modification: For knee injuries, see Standing Leg Flexion (p. 138).

Advanced Challenge: Raise your legs so that your feet and knees are about two inches off the mat. Kick the left heel to the right buttock, stretching the right leg back. Keep your feet off the mat throughout the entire exercise.

Benefit for Sports: Prevent knee injury; coordination.

Transition: Lie face down on the mat for the Double Leg Kick.

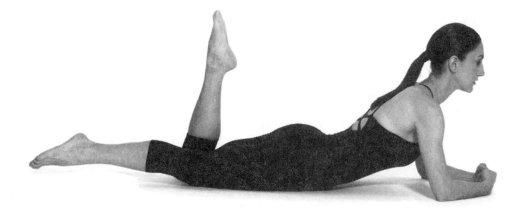

Double Leg Kick (Mobility/Strength)

- Lie on your stomach and turn your head to one side, placing your cheek on the mat. Bring your arms behind your back, clasping your hands between your shoulder blades, with your elbows touching the mat.

- Exhale. With your legs together, kick the buttocks three times.

- After the third kick, with your legs straight on the mat, engage your powerhouse as you lift your upper body off the mat. Open your chest and reach your hands straight back to your feet. Inhale.

- Repeat 2 times on each side.

Tip: At the end of the movement, as you stretch backward, remember to keep your feet on the mat and reach long through the top of the head.

Modification: For stiff shoulders, keep your arms by your sides.

Benefit for Sports: Invert the spine; spinal flexibility for cycling.

Transition: Sit back on your heels to open the lower back, making sure the stomach does not touch your thighs (Spine Stretch Release). Turn over to lie on your back for the Neck Pull.

intermediate

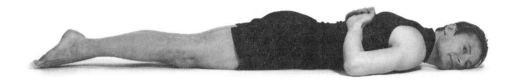

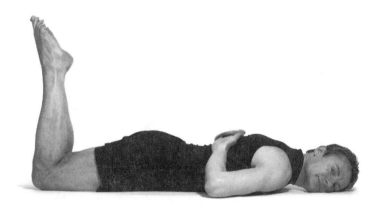

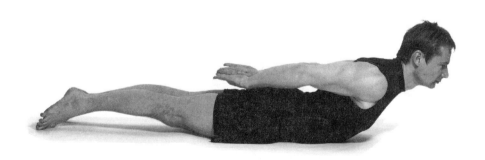

Neck Pull (Strength)

- Lie on your back with your hands placed at the base of your head and your elbows wide to the sides. Flex your feet and place them hip-width apart.

- Begin rolling up by drawing the abdominal muscles in, raising your head, and bringing your chin to your chest. Inhale. Lift your shoulders, then the upper body all the way up. Bend forward over your legs.

- Exhale, bringing your head to your knees, all the while your stomach is lifting in and up.

- Inhale as you roll up your spine to a sitting position, elbows still open wide, keeping a long neck and a straight spine.

- Start to roll back by sliding your tailbone under you. Use your powerhouse to push your spine into the mat all the way down, one vertebra at a time, exhaling.

- Repeat 5 times.

Tip: Slide your shoulder blades down toward your hips. Dig your heels into the mat when rolling up, and flex your feet as you roll down. Do not put pressure on your head while rolling up.

Modification: If you are unable to roll up with straight legs, slightly bend your knees. You may also keep your arms by your sides.

Advanced Challenge: Keep your spine straight and lean back as far as you can go, maintaining a straight back before rolling down to finish.

Benefit for Sports: Prevent lower back injury; spinal stability.

Transition: Intermediate go to Side Kick Series, Advanced go to Jack Knife.

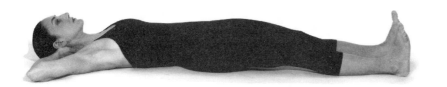

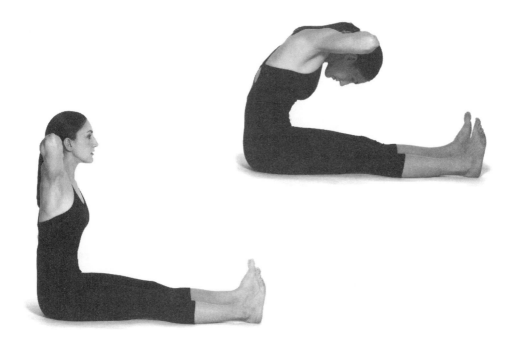

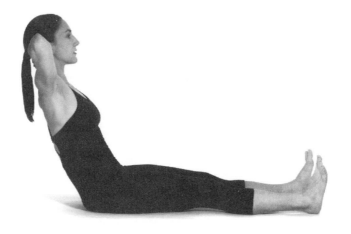

Jack Knife (Strength/Control)

- Lying on your back, bring your legs straight up to 90 degrees. Place your feet in Pilates stance and your arms by your sides.

- Inhale and engage the powerhouse, lift your buttocks to raise your legs up and overhead so they are at a 45-degree angle to the floor.

- Immediately straighten your legs so your toes are pointing toward the ceiling.

- Roll down your spine, exhaling, controlling the movement with your stomach, until your tailbone reaches the mat.

- Bring your legs back to a 90-degree angle.

- Repeat 3 times.

Tip: It is important not to go too slowly on the way down so as not to strain your back or put pressure on the neck. Keep your feet over your eyes while rolling down.

Benefit for Sports: Reverse blood flow; release tension.

Transition: Keep your legs together and sit up tall for the Spine Twist.

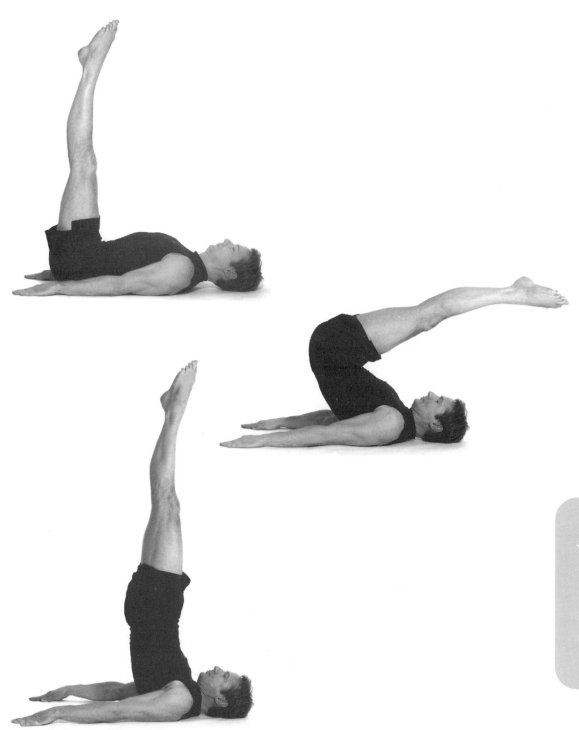

Spine Twist (Mobility)

- Sitting up tall with your legs together and your feet flexed, stretch your arms out to the sides, shoulder height.

- Inhale as you lift taller by lifting out of your hips. Twist twice to one side as you exhale. Return to center.

- Repeat 3 times on each side, remembering to use the power-house to lift your torso as tall as possible.

Tip: Heels must stay together to keep your hips stable while twisting. Work from the waist and not from the arms, and look behind you as you twist.

Benefit for Sports: Torso rotation for golf and tennis.

Transition: Lie down on your back with your knees into your chest for the Shoulder Stand Scissors.

advanced

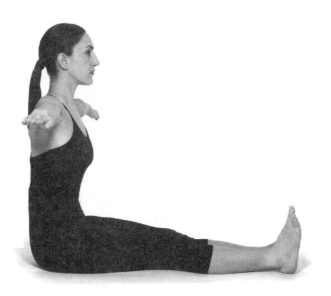

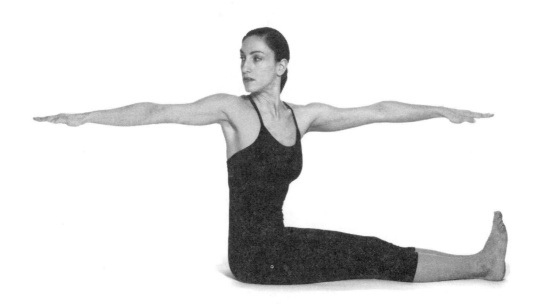

Shoulder Stand Scissors
(Mobility/Control)

- Lying on your back, bring your knees into your chest and lift your legs overhead as you lift your torso up off the mat. With your elbows on the mat, support your hips with your hands.

- Straighten your legs to the ceiling and inhale. Scissor your legs in the air, keeping them straight. Exhale. Try to lower your legs as low to the floor in front of you as possible, like you are doing a split.

- Repeat 5 sets.

Tip: Try to keep your elbows in line with your shoulders for better stability. The focus is on the leg that is reaching down in front of you.

Benefit for Sports: Recovery of tired legs for running and cycling.

Transition: Keep your lower body lifted and hips up for the Shoulder Stand Bicycle.

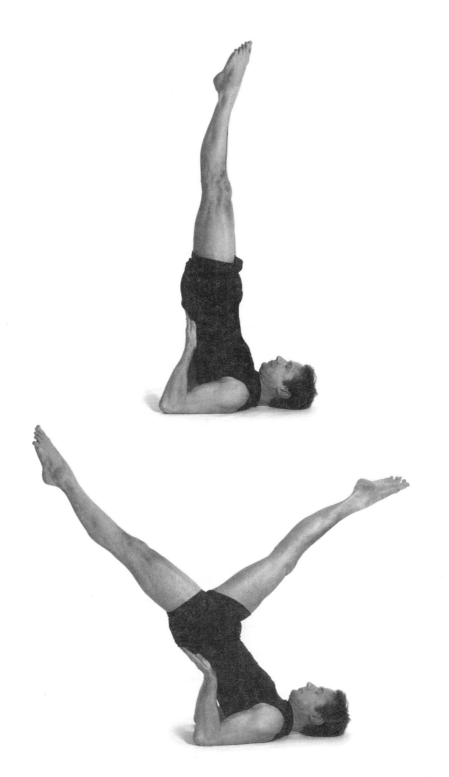

SHOULDER STAND SCISSORS

Shoulder Stand Bicycle

(Mobility/Control)

- From the Shoulder Stand Scissors position, bicycle your legs in a large circular motion.

- Following the movement of one of your legs, inhale as you bend the knee, exhale as you stretch the leg.

- Repeat 5 times then reverse the movement 5 times.

Tip: Try to keep your body supported with your shoulders and elbows to relieve pressure on the neck, and keep your legs reaching away from your chest.

Benefit for Sports: Recovery of tired legs for running and cycling.

Transition: Bend your knees into your chest and roll down your spine for the Shoulder Bridge.

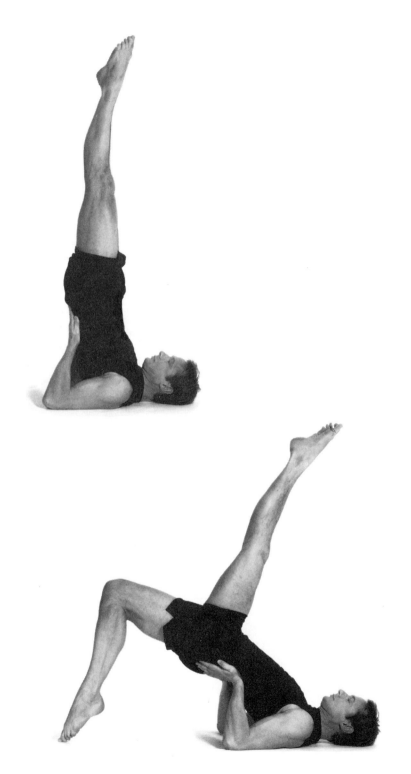

Shoulder Bridge (Strength/Mobility)

- Lying down on your back with your knees bent and feet flat on the mat, hip-distance apart, lift your buttocks up. Support your hips with your hands, with your elbows and upper arms on the mat.

- Inhale. Straighten the right leg up, pointing your toe, and then flex your foot as you lower it to knee level. Exhale.

- Repeat 3 times then switch legs.

Tip: Remember to keep your hips square throughout the exercise by engaging your powerhouse, especially when you lower your leg.

Modification: For shoulder, back, elbow, wrist, and knee injuries, see Pelvic Curl (p. 286).

Advanced Challenge: Keep your arms flat on the mat instead of using them to elevate your hips.

Benefit for Sports: Pelvic and hip stability for skiing and running.

Transition: Roll down your spine until you are flat on your back. Turn onto one side for the Side Kick Series.

advanced

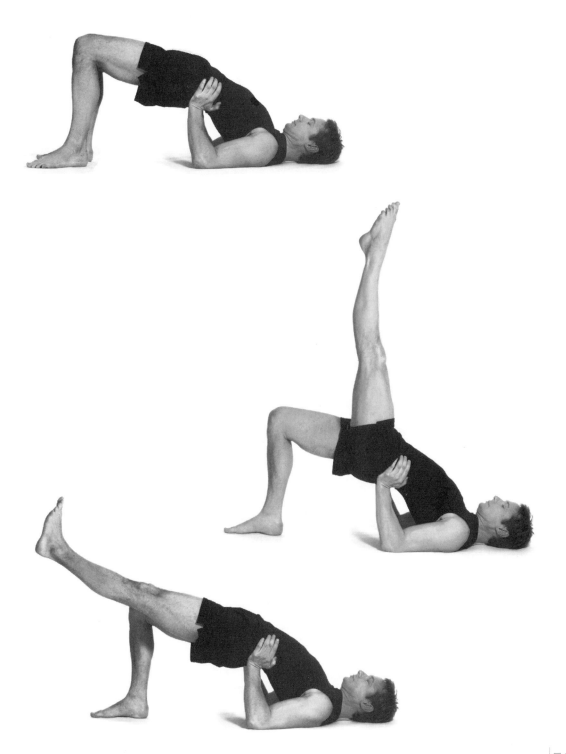

Side Kick Series

Lie down on your side, lining up your body with the back edge of the mat. Rest your head on your hand, with the other hand resting on the mat in front of your stomach. Bring your legs in front of you at a 45-degree angle (home position). Engage your powerhouse to keep the upper body still and the hips stacked on top of each other throughout the exercises. Concentrate on stabilizing your spine with your abdominal muscles to move your legs more easily. Your leg movements should be flowing and smooth. Do the full series on one side then switch to other side.

Side Kick Series: Front/Back
(Mobility)

- Keeping your legs straight, lift the top leg to hip height. Slightly rotate the leg outward from the hip (with your knee turned toward the ceiling).

- Inhale. Engage your abdominal muscles and make a big kick and pulse twice to the front.

- Exhale. Stretch the leg long to the back.

- The kick front should be loose but controlled, while you should stretch the leg long on the back kick.

- Repeat 5 to 10 times.

Tip: Keep your leg the same height throughout the exercise and keep your hips and shoulders stacked on top of each other. Do no allow your upper body to move.

Modification: For a tired neck, place your head on an outstretched arm or cushion.

Advanced Challenge: Bring your top hand behind your head.

Benefit for Sports: Hip stability and flexibility; agility; recovery of tired legs especially for tennis, running, and cycling.

Transition: Bring your legs together in home position.

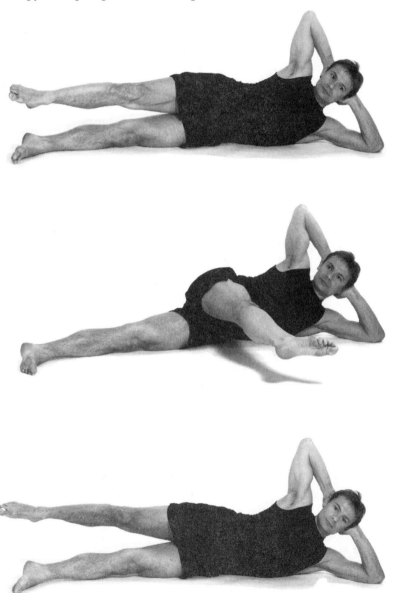

Side Kick Series: Up/Down
(Strength)

- Inhale. Kick your leg up to the ceiling with energy.

- Lengthen your leg from the hip as it reaches down to home position, resisting against gravity with your inner thigh. Exhale.

- Repeat 5 times.

Tip: Reach your leg out from your hip joint as you lower to lengthen the leg and keep your top hip reaching away from your rib cage.

Modification: For a tired neck, place your head on an outstretched arm or cushion.

Advanced Challenge: Bring your top hand behind your head.

Benefit for Sports: Work lateral stabilizer muscles for skiing, running, and cycling.

Transition: Bring your legs together in home position.

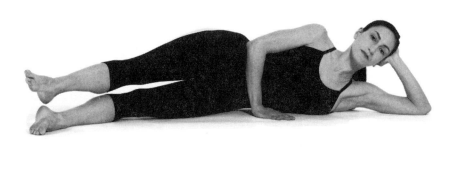

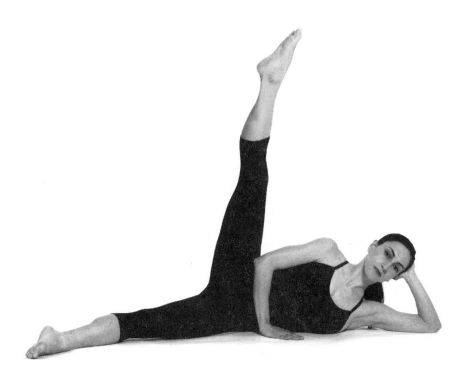

Side Kick Series: Small Circles
(Mobility)

- Lift your top leg up to hip height.

- Reaching long from the hip with your leg turned out, make small circles from the hip joint.

- Repeat 5 times then reverse.

Tip: Lengthen the leg out of the hip. Make circles with your whole leg, not just your foot.

Modification: For a tired neck, place your head on an outstretched arm or cushion.

Benefit for Sports: Hip joint flexibility.

Transition: Intermediate go to Teaser 1, Advanced bring your legs together in home position.

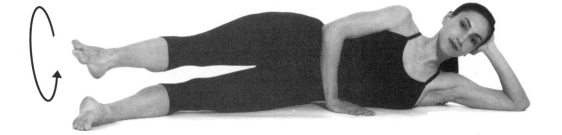

Side Kick Series: Bicycle (Mobility)

- Lift the top leg up to hip height. Inhale, kick the top leg to the front.

- Bicycle the top leg, bending it in front of your body and extending it straight behind you.

- Repeat 3 times, then reverse the bicycle.

Tip: Lengthen the leg out of the hip. Keep your hips and shoulders stacked on top of each other. Do not allow your upper body to move.

Modification: For a tired neck, place your head on an outstretched arm or cushion.

Advanced Challenge: Bring your top hand behind your head.

Benefit for Sports: Postural strength; hip joint flexibility.

Transition: Bring your legs together in home position.

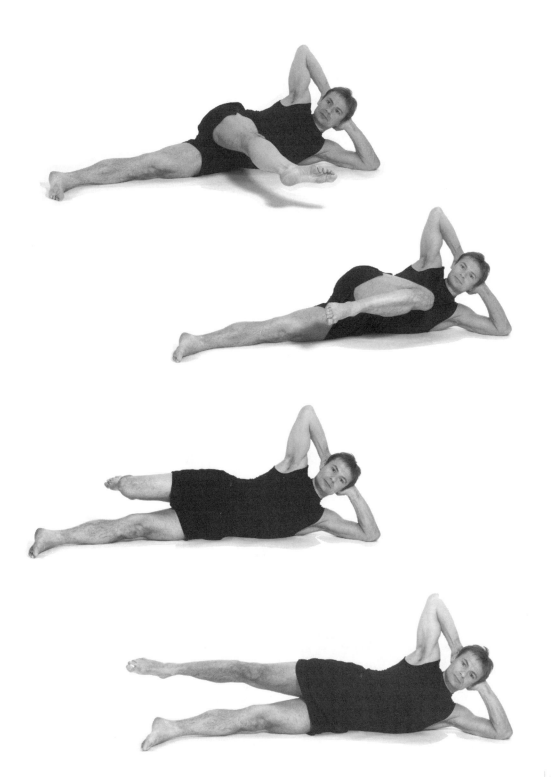

Side Kick Series: Double Leg Lift

(Strength)

- With your legs together, inhale and lift them both up 2 to 5 inches from the ground. Hold for 3 counts.

- Exhale as you lower your legs.

- Repeat 3 times.

- On the third repetition, keep the top leg up and still as you lower and lift your bottom leg 10 times.

Tip: Keep the powerhouse engaged and your hips aligned and lift your waist.

Modification: For a tired neck, place your head on an outstretched arm or cushion.

Advanced Challenge: Try to keep both hands behind your head.

Benefit for Sports: Postural strength; works lateral stabilizer muscles, which is especially good for skiing, running, and cycling.

Transition: Bring your legs together in home position.

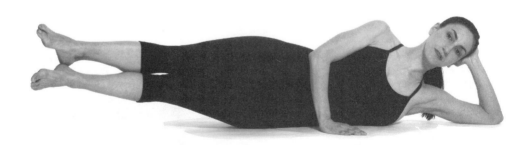

advanced

Side Kick Series: Inner Thigh Lift

(Strength)

- Bend your top leg and cross it in front of the bottom leg by placing the foot flat on the floor directly in front of your bottom thigh.

- Hold on to the ankle from the inside of your leg. Lift the bottom leg, making sure to keep your hips stacked on top of each other so that they do not roll back.

- Make big circles 5 times in each direction, then reverse.

Tip: Lift from the inner thigh and reach the leg long from the hip.

Modification: For a tired neck, place your head on an outstretched arm or cushion.

Benefit for Sports: Work medial stabilizer muscles in skiing, cycling, swimming, and running.

Transition: Bring the legs together in home position.

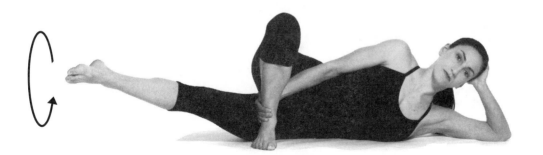

Side Kick Series: Hot Potato

(Strength)

- Lightly tap the heel of the top foot in front of the other foot 5 times.

- Kick the top leg up to the ceiling then lower it to touch the mat behind the bottom foot. Tap it 5 times.

- Kick the top leg and tap in front of the bottom foot 4 times. Continue to tap and lift, decreasing the amount of taps by one each time.

- When you reach 1 (your foot should be in back), lift and tap once in front, then once in back and repeat.

Tip: Keep dynamic energy in the leg while kicking.

Modification: For a tired neck, place your head on an outstretched arm or cushion.

Benefit for Sports: Work lateral stabilizer muscles for skiing, running, and cycling.

Transition: Bring your legs together in the home position.

advanced

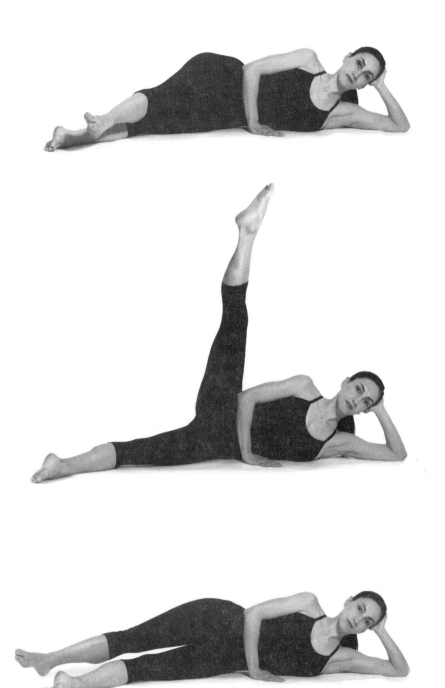

Side Kick Series: Big Scissors

(Control/Mobility)

- Lift both legs off the mat about 2 inches, keeping one hand in front of you on the mat for stability.

- Kick one leg front and the other leg back, making a big scissors with your straight legs.

- Repeat 5 to 10 times.

Tip: Keep your powerhouse engaged and hips aligned.

Benefit for Sports: Hip flexibility; postural strength in the torso.

Transition: Bring your legs together in home position.

advanced

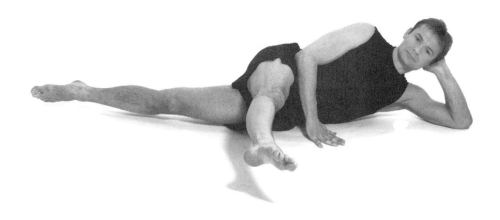

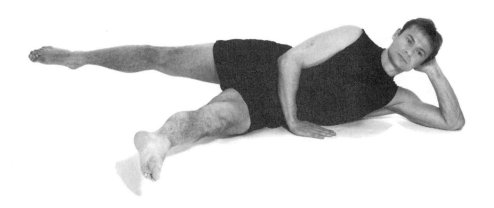

Side Kick Series: Ronde de Jambe

(Mobility/Control/Strength)

- Kick your top leg straight to the front.

- Lift it outward up to the ceiling.

- Rotate the leg out from the hip, then continue the outward movement as you reach it back behind you.

- Complete the large circle by returning to home position.

- Repeat 3 times.

- Reverse by kicking the leg back, lifting it up to the ceiling, rotating out, and bringing it around to the front and then home.

- Repeat 3 times.

Tip: Keep the legs long and soft (not tense). Use the opposite energy of your hips reaching away from the top of your head and your working leg reaching away from your hips.

Modification: For a tired neck, place your head on an outstretched arm or cushion.

Advanced Challenge: Bring your top hand behind your head.

Benefit for Sports: Increase range of motion in the hip joint.

Transition: Roll onto your stomach for the Transition/Leg Beats. Or, when you have completed both legs in the Side Kick Series, go to Teaser 1.

advanced

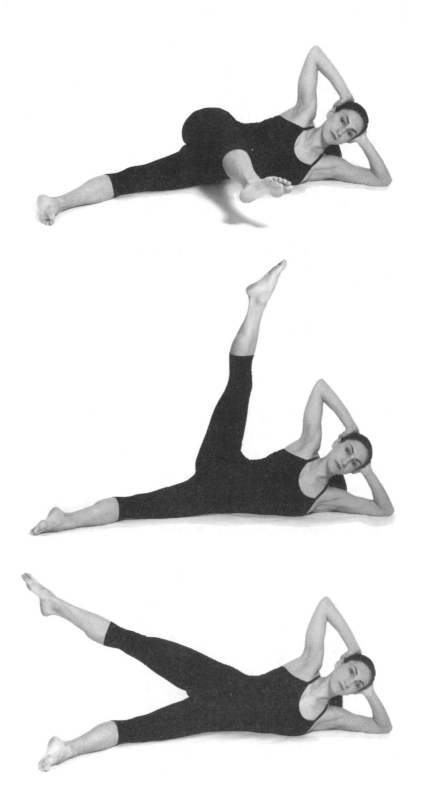

Side Kick Series: Transition/Leg Beats (Strength)

- Turn onto your stomach, placing your head on your hands. Your hands should be palms down on the mat with your elbows stretched out to your sides.

- Relax your upper body and engage (lift) your abdominal muscles.

- With your feet in Pilates stance, lift straight legs 2 inches off the mat and beat your inner thighs together.

- Repeat 10 to 20 times.

Tip: Keep your abdominal muscles lifted to support your lower back.

Benefit for Sports: Postural strength for the lower back.

Transition: Roll over onto your other side and repeat the entire Side Kick Series with the other leg. You will not repeat this exercise a second time. When you have completed both legs, continue on to Teaser 1.

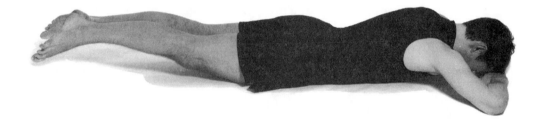

Teaſer 1 (Strength/Control)

- Lie down on your back.

- Straighten your arms and extend them over your head up by your ears. Lift your legs to a 45-degree angle, keeping your entire spine on the mat.

- Bring your head up and your chin to your chest. Inhale and roll up to reach for your toes. Balance on your sitting bones, holding the position and lifting your stomach and lower back.

- Keep your fingers reaching for your toes and exhale as you roll back down to the floor with control, keeping your legs at a 45-degree angle.

- Repeat 3 times.

Tip: Press your stomach to your spine when initiating the movement and press your lower back into the mat when you are reclined.

Modification: If you have difficulty holding your feet up, try slightly bending the knees, while keeping the toes higher than the knees.

Benefit for Sports: Balance; concentration.

Transition: Intermediate go to Seal, Advanced go to Teaser 2.

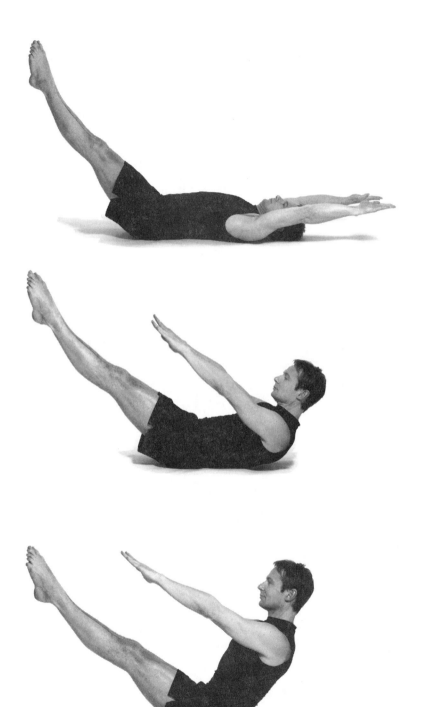

Teaser 2 (Control/Strength)

- Begin with the first 3 steps of Teaser 1. Reach for your toes and hold the position, balancing on your sitting bones.

- Keeping your upper body perfectly still, lower and lift your legs 3 times. Exhale as you lower the legs, inhale as you lift them.

- Finish by lifting your arms over your head. Roll your entire body all the way down with your arms remaining next to your ears.

Tip: Keep your torso lifted and straight.

Benefit for Sports: Balance; concentration; stabilize the torso.

Transition: Roll your entire body down to the mat, vertebra by vertebra, with your feet touching the mat simultaneously with the head. You are ready for Teaser 3.

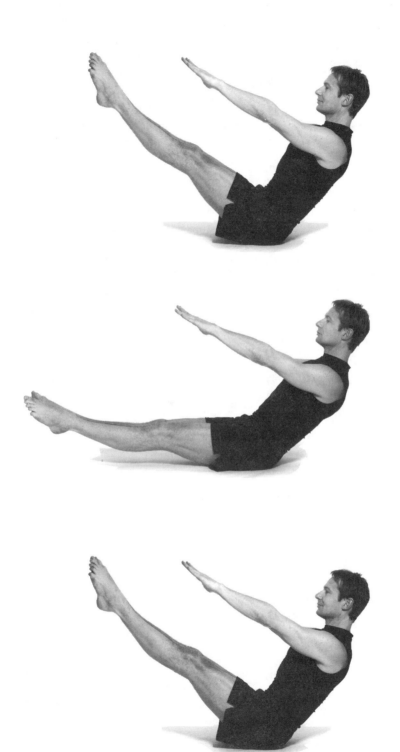

TEASER 2

Teaser 3 (Strength/Control)

- Lie down with your arms stretched up by your ears and your feet on the floor.

- Inhale. Engage the powerhouse and roll your entire body up to a "V" position, balancing on your sitting bones.

- Reach for your toes and then lift your arms to the ceiling. Hold the position, then roll your entire body down slowly with control. Exhale. Your heels and head should touch the mat simultaneously.

- Repeat 3 times.

Tip: Use the powerhouse to bring your body up without using your legs or momentum to get you there. Try to feel the resistance of your arms and legs reaching in opposite directions, which lengthens your spine.

Benefit for Sports: Balance; control.

Transition: Sit up with your legs straight out in front of you on the mat for the Boomerang.

advanced

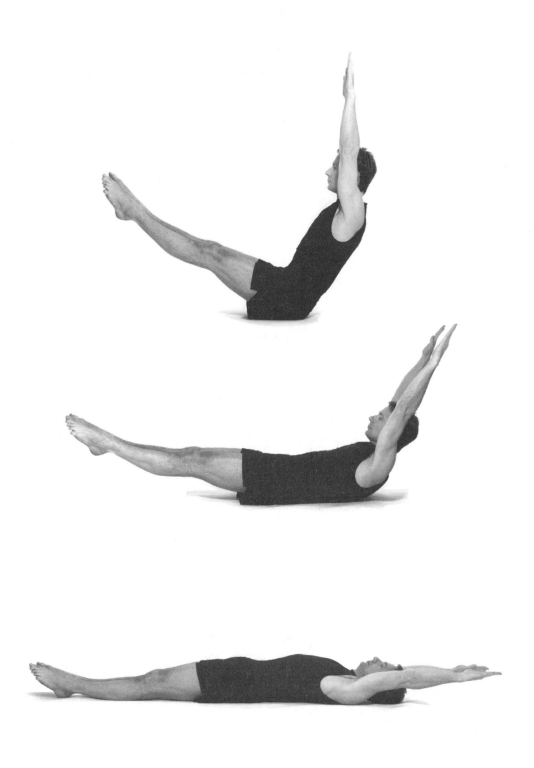

Boomerang (Control)

- Sit up tall with your legs straight out in front of you and your right ankle crossed over the left. Place your hands palms down next to your hips on the mat.

- Inhale. Lift your feet and roll back gently, bringing your legs overhead until they are parallel to the floor.

- While your legs are overhead, open them shoulder-width apart and then close them, placing the left ankle over the right.

- Roll up into a Teaser position, reaching for your toes and keeping your legs at a 45-degree angle. Exhale.

- Bend your arms by your sides and reach them behind your back, maintaining the Teaser position.

- Clasp your hands behind your back, inhale, and stretch them upward. Unclasp your hands and open your arms as you circle them over your head to reach your toes again, rolling the whole body forward.

- Gently roll your whole body forward, stretching over your legs. Exhale.

- Roll up to sitting/home position.

- Repeat 4 times, switching legs each time.

Tip: Keep your powerhouse lifted as you reach for the toes to get the full stretch. The entire movement should be controlled by abdominal strength and executed smoothly.

Advanced Challenge: After rolling to the Teaser position, bend your arms by your sides and circle them around to reach for your toes again. Using control from your powerhouse, lower your upper body and legs at the same time, all the way to the floor. Stretch forward.

Benefit for Sports: Dynamic balance.

Transition: Place your arms behind you on the mat for Hip Circles.

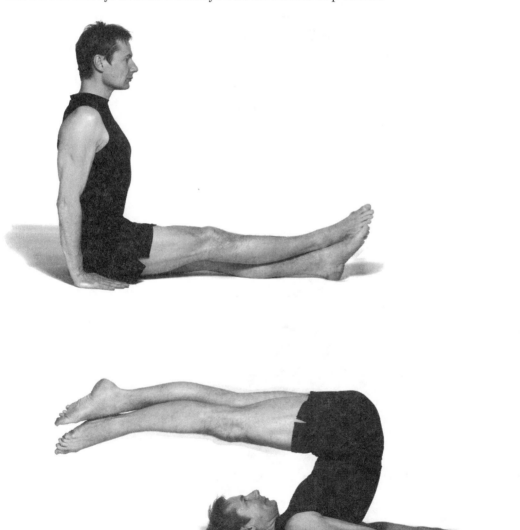

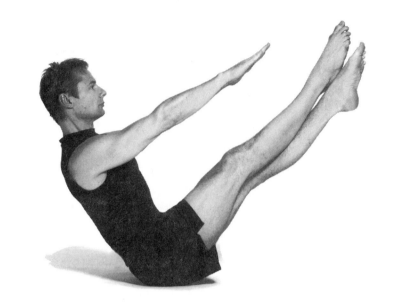

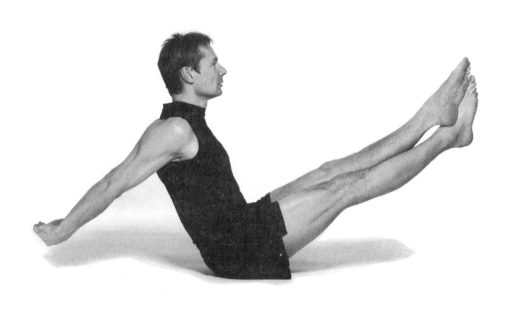

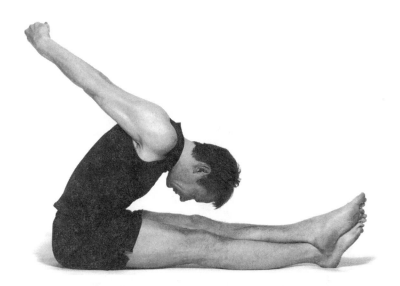

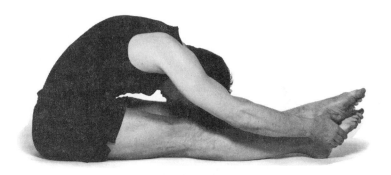

Hip Circles (Strength)

- Sit up tall with straight arms behind you resting on the mat. Lift your legs and keep your body in a "V" position.

- Inhale. Keeping your feet in Pilates stance, make a big circle with your legs around to the right side, down, and back up to the left and center. Exhale.

- Reverse the circle.

- Repeat 3 sets.

Tip: Make sure to keep your chest open and your back and arms straight, lengthening your neck out of your shoulders.

Modification: For back pain, omit the exercise, or you can try doing the exercise with your forearms on the mat.

Advanced Challenge: Try to bring your legs up to touch your nose.

Benefit for Sports: Torso rotation.

Transition: Roll onto your stomach for Swimming.

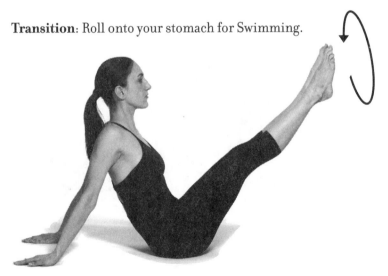

Swimming (Strength)

- On your stomach, stretch your arms out in front of you and your legs long behind you.

- Raise your right arm and left leg, lift your head.

- Begin to kick your legs up and down as you pump your arms up and down.

- Breath to a count of 5 (like the Hundred, p. 24), inhaling for 5 counts through the nose, and exhaling for 5 counts through the mouth.

- Do 2 sets of 10 repetitions—inhale on 5, exhale on 5.

Tip: Keep the powerhouse engaged while on your stomach.

Modification: For a sore neck, rest your forehead on your hands and kick the legs as stated above.

Benefit for Sports: Prevent lower back pain; stabilize lumbar spine; prevent kyphosis.

Transition: Sit back on your heels to open your lower back (Spine Stretch Release). Bring your body into a push-up position.

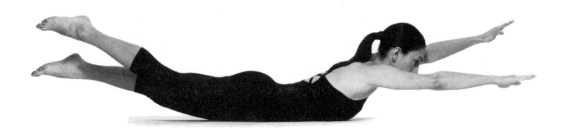

SWIMMING

Leg Pull Down (Strength)

- Lying on your stomach, bring your body into a push-up position, with your feet in Pilates stance and your wrists lined up directly below your shoulders.

- Inhale. Lift the right leg up straight out behind you. Stretch the supporting heel backward, letting your weight shift backward and then forward. Exhale.

- Switch to the left foot.

- Repeat 3 sets on each leg.

Tip: Your powerhouse controls the body, keeping it in a straight line. Make sure to keep your hips even.

Modification: When you do this movement for the first time, you may want to try it on your forearms.

Benefit for Sports: Ankle flexibility; balance; postural strength; control.

Transition: Sit back on your heels (Spine Stretch Release) and turn over for the Leg Pull Up.

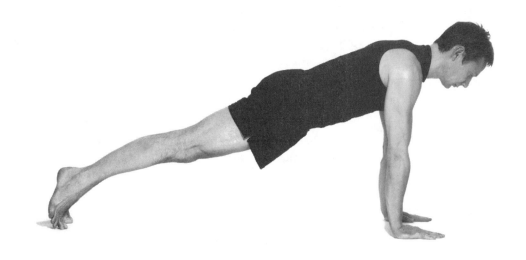

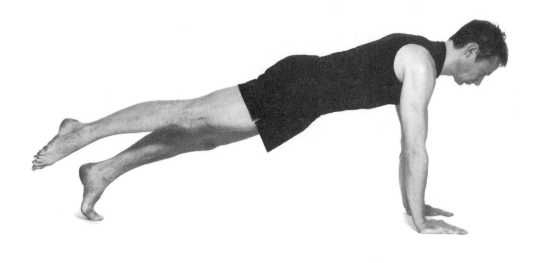

Leg Pull Up (Strength)

- From a sitting position with straight legs and your hands by your hips, lift your hips up to make your body a straight diagonal line from your shoulders to your heels. Keep your weight on the outer edges of your feet.

- Inhale. Keeping your chin to your chest, kick one leg up to the ceiling, pointing your toes to reach your nose.

- Exhale as you bring the flexed leg back down. Switch legs.

- Repeat 3 times, alternating legs.

Tip: Your wrists should be in line with your shoulders. Keep your hips lifted and even as the leg kicks up.

Modification: Keep one leg bent at a 90-degree angle with the foot on the floor.

Benefit for Sports: Postural and dynamic strength.

Transition: Kneel on both knees for Kneeling Side Kicks.

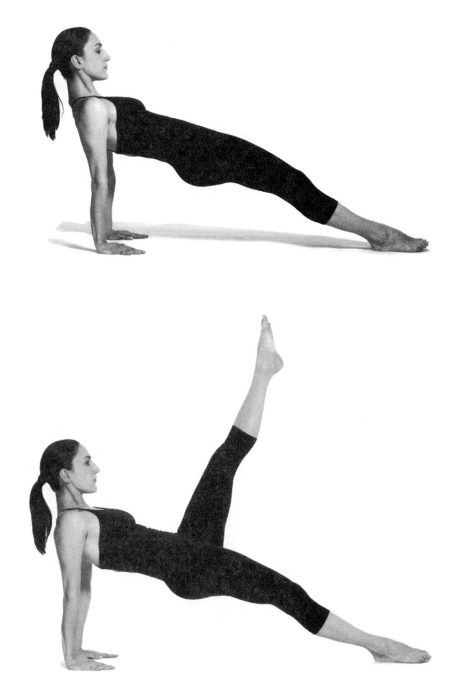

Kneeling Side Kicks (Control)

- From a kneeling position, bend your torso at the waist to place your right hand on the mat directly below your shoulder.

- Raise the left leg straight out from your hip until it is hip level.

- Inhale. Kick your leg to the front of your body, then stretch it long to the back. Exhale. Keep the leg hip height throughout the exercise.

- Repeat 5 times. Kneel on both knees then switch to the other leg.

Tip: Make sure to keep your hip lifted and the long leg reaching out. The body should stay stable as only the leg moves.

Benefit for Sports: Correct imbalances; dynamic balance; isolate hip joint for skiing.

Transition: Sit on the mat with your legs in front of you to prepare for the Mermaid.

advanced

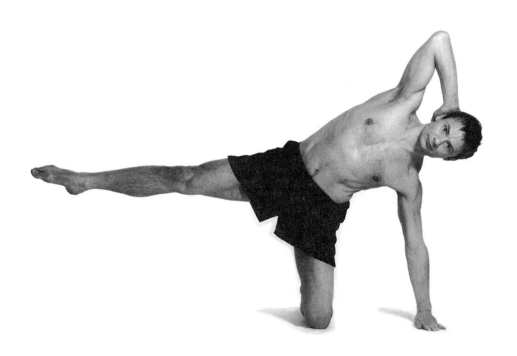

Mermaid (Mobility)

- From a seated position on the mat, bend your legs and curl them to the right, tucking your feet close to your buttocks so that your weight is on your right hip. Hold on to your ankles with your left hand and lift your right arm next to your head.

- Inhale. Stretch up and over to the left, bending your right elbow to round your arm so that it touches your left ear. Exhale. Straighten your arm and lift your body back to center.

- Inhale. Bring the right forearm down to the mat to support yourself as you lift and stretch your left arm up to your ear and over to the right. Exhale.

- Repeat 3 times then turn on to your left hip and repeat 3 times, stretching further out to the side each time.

Tip: Remember to lift from your center and stretch the sides, keeping your ribs in.

Modification: For knee injuries, do the Arm Weights Series: Side to Side (p. 146).

Benefit for Sports: Improve lateral flexibility in the torso; release tension in the shoulders and upper back.

Transition: Sit on your right hip with your legs slightly bent to the side for the Snake.

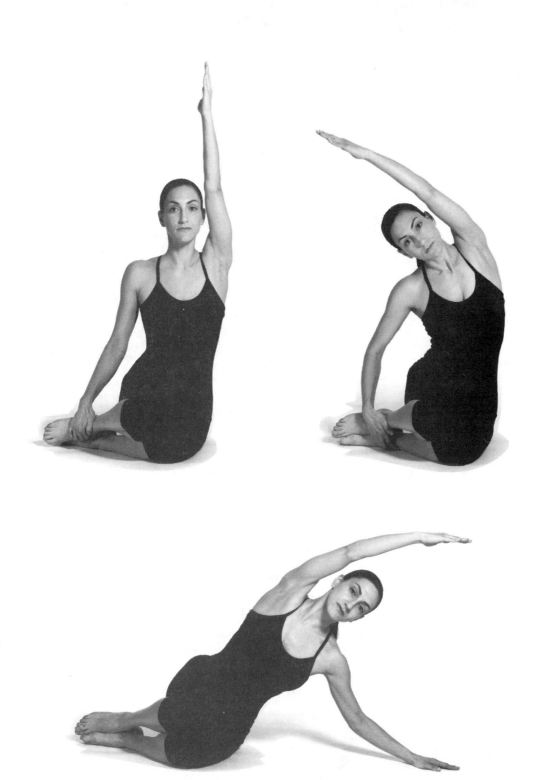

Snake (Strength/Control)

- Sitting on your right hip with your legs in front of you, slightly bend your knees and place the left heel just in front of your right foot.

- Place your right hand on the mat in line with your shoulder and hip. Place your left hand on the mat just in front of your upper body.

- Inhale, lift the hips, and turn your hips and shoulders toward the mat as you rise up onto your toes.

- Exhale and lower your hips toward the mat and arch your back. Lift your chest to the ceiling.

- Inhale and bring the hips up once again by using your power-house.

- Exhale and bend the knees and lower your body down to the starting position.

- Repeat 3 times on each side.

Tip: When coming up on your toes, make sure to lengthen both sides of the waist and keep your hips square.

Benefit for Sports: Invert the spine; prevent kyphosis; improve breathing.

Transition: Sit back down on your right hip for Twist 1.

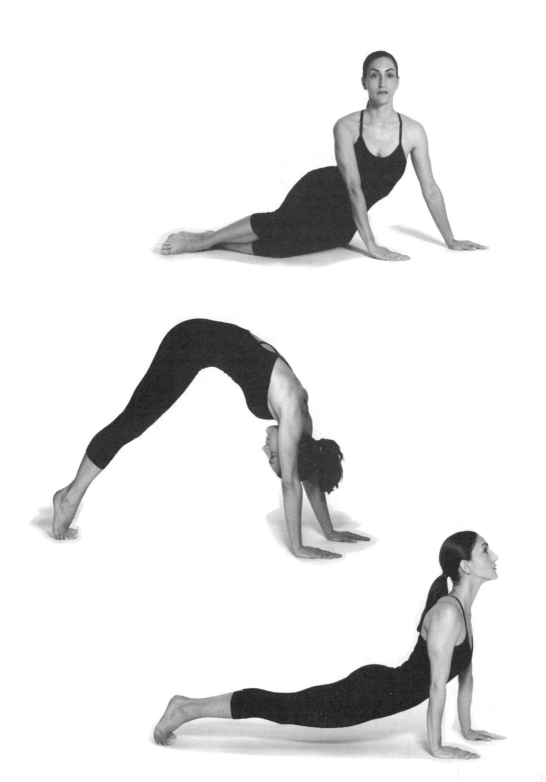

Twist 1 (Mobility/Strength)

- Sit on your right hip with your legs extended and knees slightly bent. Cross your left foot just in front of the right. Place your right arm straight under your shoulder so that your wrist and shoulder are in alignment. Rest your outstretched arm on the left leg.

- Inhale as you lift your hips to make a straight diagonal line with your body. Raise your left arm above your head and close to your ear.

- Lower your hips close to the mat without touching it and without bending your supporting arm. Lower your left arm to your side and look down at your feet. Exhale.

- Inhale and lift your hips again.

- Exhale as you return to the starting position.

- Repeat 3 times on each side.

Tip: Keep your hips lifted and place an equal amount of pressure on your bottom heel and hand. The control in this exercise initiates from the powerhouse, especially the obliques.

Benefit for Sports: Balance; torso stabilization; postural strength, especially for the sides.

Transition: Sit on your right hip with your legs extended and knees slightly bent for Twist 2.

advanced

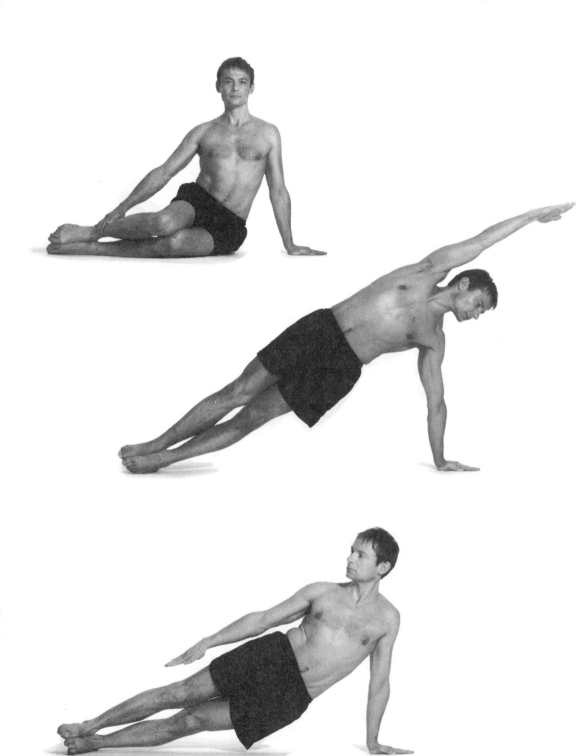

Twist 2 (Control)

- Sit on your right hip with your legs extended and your knees slightly bent. Cross your left foot just in front of the right. Place your right arm straight under your shoulder so that your wrist and shoulder are in alignment. Rest your outstretched arm on the left leg.

- Inhale as you lift your hips to make a straight diagonal line with your body. Raise your left arm above your head and close to your ear.

- Twist your body to face the mat. Lift your stomach and hips and scoop your left arm under your body. Exhale.

- Inhale. Twist your body back to facing side. Continuing the motion of your arm, raise it up the side of your body to your ear and stretch behind you.

- Follow the movement of your arm with your eyes and turn your head to look behind you. Keep your arm by your ear and lift your chest to the ceiling.

- Come back to center and gently lower your body to home position. Exhale.

- Repeat 2 times on each side.

Tip: Keep your hips lifted throughout the exercise. The control in this exercise initiates from the powerhouse, especially the obliques.

Benefit for Sports: Balance; torso stabilization; postural strength, especially for the sides.

Transition: Lie on your stomach for Rocking.

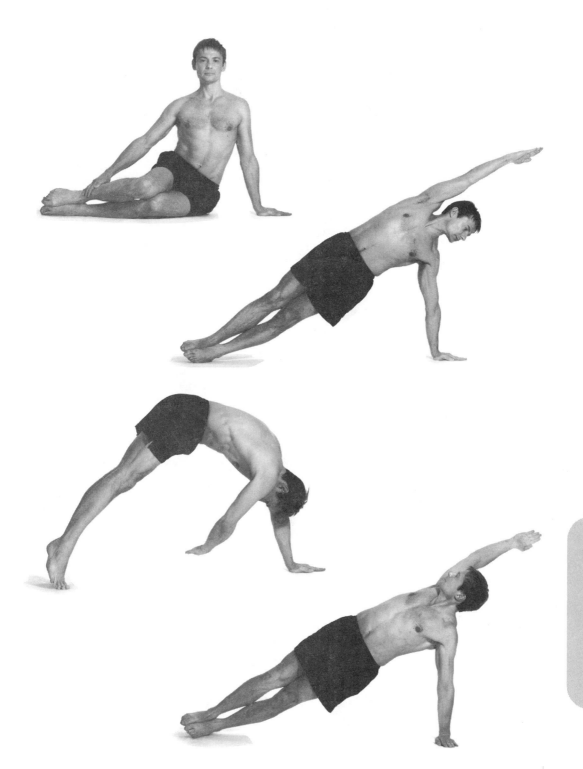

TWIST 2

Rocking (Mobility)

- Lie on your stomach, bend your knees, and reach back to grab your ankles, keeping your knees and feet together.

- With your arms, pull (stretch) your feet up to the ceiling and lift and lower the knees 3 times.

- Continuing to hold your ankles, begin to rock back (inhaling) and forth (exhaling) on your chest, using your powerhouse to initiate and control the movement.

- Repeat 6 times.

Tip: Be sure to keep your head and neck still and to keep your head and knees up while rocking. Lift your chest and knees off the mat throughout the exercise.

Benefit for Sports: Inverts the spine; prevents kyphosis, especially for cyclists.

Transition: Sit back on your heels to open your lower back. Turn over and sit up for the Crab.

advanced

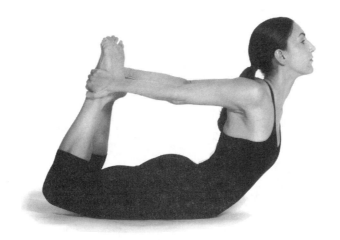

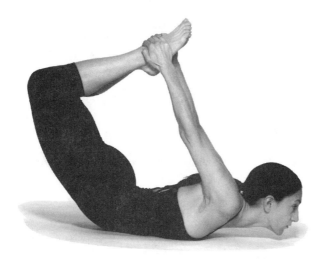

Crab (Mobility)

- Sit cross-legged at the center of the mat. Hold on to your feet and bring your knees to your shoulders. Your arms should be on the outside of your knees.

- Lean forward and rock up onto your knees as you bring your buttocks up in the air. Gently touch the top of your head to the mat, stretching your neck.

- Inhale. Roll backward onto your shoulders, bringing your legs overhead.

- While your legs are overhead, uncross your legs, opening your knees to the sides. Bring them back together, crossing them with the opposite leg on top.

- Exhale. Roll back up and forward so your head touches the floor again in front of you.

- Repeat 6 times.

Tip: Make sure to draw your abdominal muscles in while rolling on top of your head to avoid too much pressure on the neck.

Benefit for Sports: Release tension in the neck and upper back; re-generate the whole body.

Transition: Roll back one more time and lie on your back with your legs to the ceiling for the Balance Control.

advanced

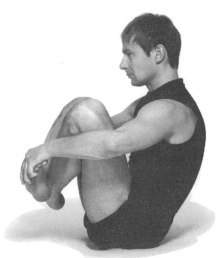

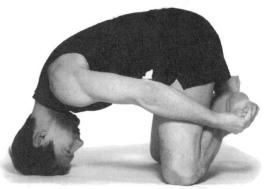

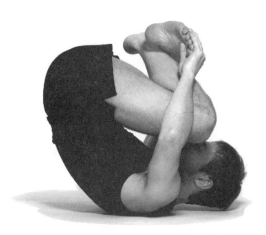

Balance Control (Control/Strength)

- Lying on your back, bring straight arms to rest on the mat above your head.

- Inhale. Lift your legs overhead until your toes touch the mat.

- Grab your right ankle with both hands and reach the left leg to the ceiling.

- Exhale. Switch legs with control, bringing the left leg down to your hands.

- Bring both legs straight into the air. Lower down gently.

- Repeat 2 sets.

Tip: Maintain balance on shoulders and keep your stomach in and back straight for better stability.

Benefit for Sports: Balance and concentration.

Transition: Roll down your spine gently and stand up for Push-up.

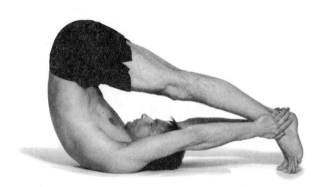

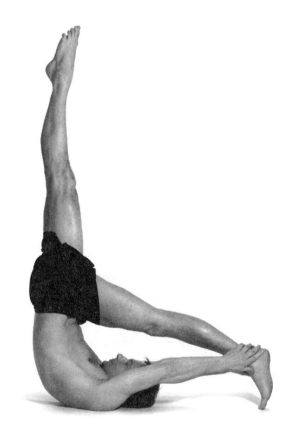

Push-up (Strength)

- Stand with your feet in Pilates stance and arms raised above your head.

- Bring your chin to your chest, engage your powerhouse, and begin to roll down your spine and lower your arms until your hands reach the floor. Keep your stomach lifted.

- With straight legs, walk your hands out on the mat until your wrists are directly below your shoulders and your body is in a straight line.

- Bending your arms backward so that your elbows point behind you, push up 3 times. Inhale when you bend your arms, exhale when you raise your body.

- When you have completed the last push-up, lift from your center by raising your hips and stomach. Walk your hands back to your feet and roll up slowly to standing, lifting arms overhead.

- Repeat 3 times.

Tip: Keep your body in one straight line by lifting the stomach and engaging the buttocks to lock your hips.

Modification: Bring your knees down to the mat for a bent-knee push-up.

Advanced Challenge: When pushing up from the mat, clap your hands. You may also clap your feet together, or clap both your hands and feet simultaneously.

Benefit for Sports: Upper body strength and control; dynamic strength.

Transition: Sit down on the mat for the Seal.

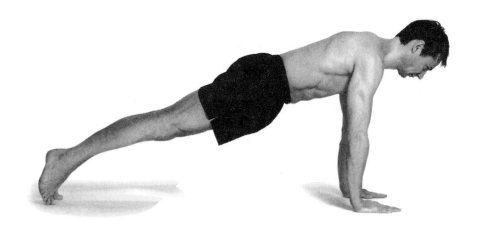

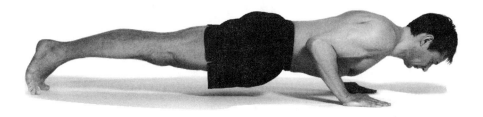

Seal (Control)

- Sit on the mat with your feet together and knees bent to the sides. Grab the outsides of your ankles by bringing your hands between your knees and under your calves. Keep the soles of your feet together.

- Sitting in a C-curve position, use your powerhouse to balance on your sitting bones. Lift your feet just off the mat and clap your feet together 3 times by opening your legs from the hips.

- Inhale. Draw your stomach in and roll back, bringing your feet overhead but keeping your head off the mat by keeping your chin to your chest. Clap 3 times with your feet overhead.

- Roll back up. Exhale. Balance on your sitting bones at the top.

- Repeat 6 times.

Tip: Keep the abdominal muscles drawn in while balancing.

Benefit for Sports: Back injury prevention; loosen hips; circulation.

Transition: On the sixth roll up, let go of your ankles, cross them, and stand up without using your arms.

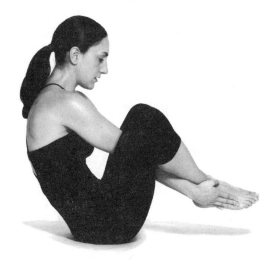

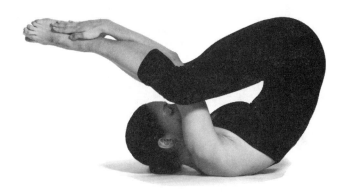

4

The Wall Series

The Wall Series exercises are intended as a cooldown (Arm Circles, Rolling Down) at the end of your workout. They are also corrective exercises for problems such as lordosis (swayback posture) (Squat), knee problems (Seated Leg Extension, Standing Leg Flexion), and exercises that help put the body back in alignment (Neck Exercise).

Arm Circles (Mobility)

- Standing with your back against a wall, place your feet in Pilates stance.

- Step your feet away from the wall, just far enough so that you're entire back remains flat against the wall, and keep your powerhouse lifted.

- Make big, loose circles with your arms, keeping them within your peripheral vision. Inhale as your arms go up and exhale as your arms come down.

- Repeat 3 to 5 times then reverse the circles.

Tip: This exercise can be done with 2- to 3-pound weights.

Benefit for Sports: Improve shoulder range of motion; prevent lordosis.

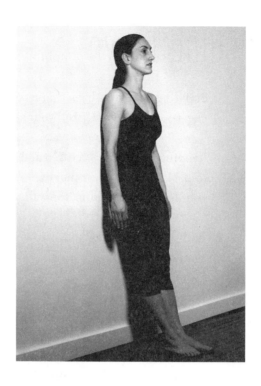

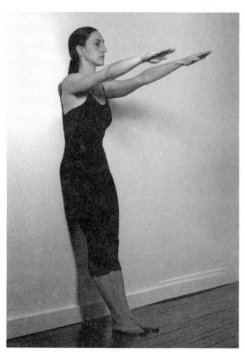

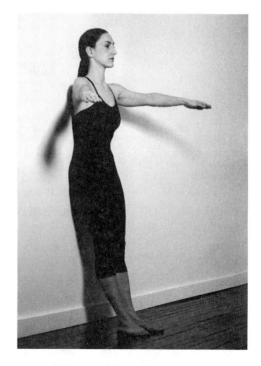

Rolling Down (Mobility)

- Standing with your back against a wall, bring your chin to your chest, and then gently roll your shoulders forward off the wall.

- Keeping your stomach lifted and pressed into your spine, start to peel off the wall, removing one vertebra at a time, keeping your lower back against the wall.

- Roll down as far as you can while keeping your lower back against the wall.

- Let your hanging arms make a few tiny, loose, effortless circles in one direction. Then reverse the direction of the circles.

- Stop the circles and let your arms hang heavy. Draw your stomach in and up, slowly rolling back up the wall, pressing each vertebra individually into the wall as you roll up to standing.

Tip: Visualize the opposition of your stomach pulling in while your spine pulls away from the wall. Keep your head and shoulders heavy and relaxed, while keeping your stomach lifted.

Advanced Challenge: This exercise can be done with 2- to 3-pound weights. You may also roll all the way down to your toes.

Benefit for Sports: Release shoulder tension; improve postural and abdominal control; prevent lordosis.

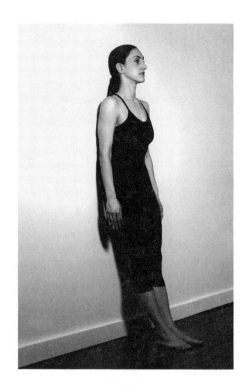

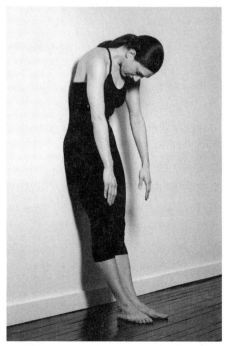

Squat (Strength)

- Standing with your back against a wall, separate your feet to hip distance apart and bring them away from the wall.

- Inhale. Lift the powerhouse and begin to slide down the wall into a sitting position. Make sure that your knees are not further forward than your feet.

- As you slide down, lift your arms so that they are parallel to your shoulders. Keep your back against the wall and hold the position for 5 counts.

- Slide back up the wall and lower your arms. Exhale.

- Repeat 3 times.

Tip: Do not go lower than a right angle with your knees.

Advanced Challenge: This exercise can be done with 2- to 3-pound weights to increase the challenge. You may also raise your arms above your head while sliding down. Hold the position until you slide back up, then lower your arms with control. Holding the position longer will also increase the challenge.

Benefit for Sports: Strength/power in lower body; postural strength; prevent back pain.

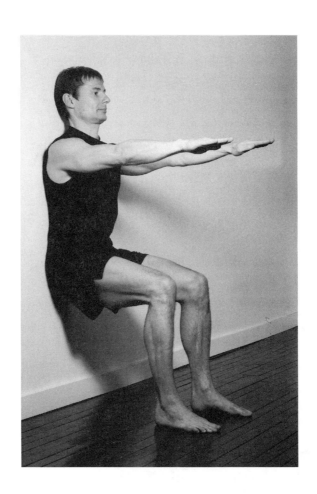

Squat One Leg (Strength/Control)

- Stand against a wall with your feet together in a parallel position and in front of you, keeping your knees together.

- Lift one leg to hip height and your arms to shoulder height as you slide down the wall.

- Hold for 3 to 5 counts, then slide back up the wall, lowering your arms and leg as you slide up.

- Repeat 2 times then switch legs.

Tip: Keep your knees together to increase stability.

Modification: See Seated Leg Extension (p. 136).

Benefit for Sports: Correct muscle imbalance in the lower body; postural strength.

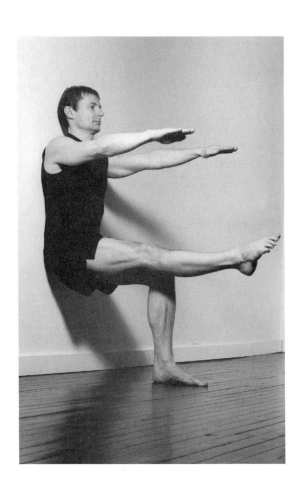

Seated Leg Extension (Strength)

- Sit on a chair with your legs at a right angle to the floor.

- Inhale and straighten one leg from the knee. Hold for 5 counts.

- Exhale and bend the knee, lower the leg, and switch legs.

- Repeat 5 times on each leg.

Tip: Make sure that the chair is the correct height—meaning that your leg is at a 90-degree angle to the floor.

Benefit for Sports: Knee-joint stability; strengthen the area surrounding the knee.

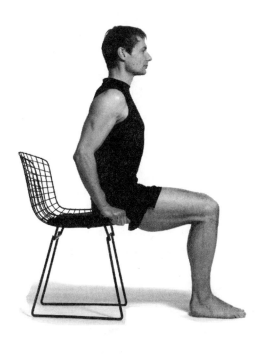

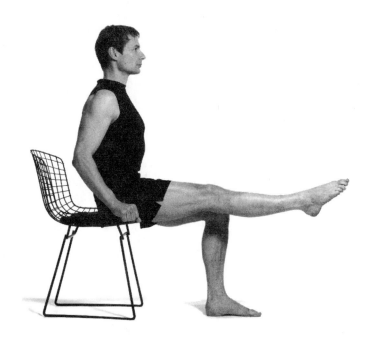

Standing Leg Flexion (Strength)

- Face a wall, outstretch your arms, and place your palms on the wall.

- Reach one leg backward, keeping your supporting leg slightly bent.

- Gently bend your extended knee and try to touch the buttocks with your heel. Hold for 10 counts.

- Lower the leg slowly with control.

- Repeat 3 times on each leg.

Tip: Keep the stomach lifted and the tailbone tucked under you (not sticking out behind you).

Benefit for Sports: Knee-joint stability.

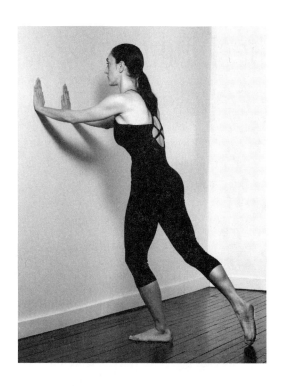

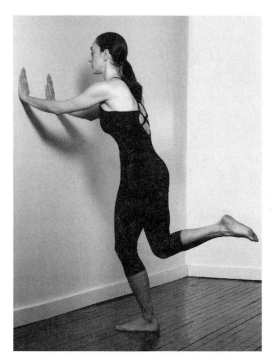

Neck Exercise (Strength)

- Stand with your back against a wall.

- Walk your feet away from the wall in Pilates stance until only the back of your head is touching the wall and your body is out at an angle.

- Hold for 10 counts.

- Walk your feet back to the wall to release.

- Walk away from the wall. Repeat 2 times.

- After 3 reps, walk your feet back to the wall and then step away, being careful not to arch your back.

Tip: Keep your neck long, shoulders relaxed, and body in one straight line.

Modification: This exercise can also be done with your hands placed behind your head instead of using the wall. With your hands overlapped and behind your head, gently press the back of your head into your hands. Hold for 5 to 10 counts. Repeat 3 times. Then put palms overlapped on your forehead and press your head into your hands. Hold 5 to 10 counts. Repeat 3 times.

Advanced Challenge: Increase the length of time you hold the position to 20 or 30 counts.

Benefit for Sports: Prevent cervical spine injury; correct poor posture.

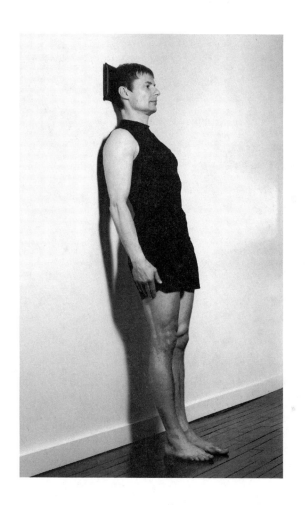

5

The Arm Weights Series

The Arm Weights Series is intended to work your powerhouse in a standing position and to help correct your posture in addition to toning your arms. Use 2- to 5-pound weights and always keep your powerhouse engaged and your weight shifted forward and up.

In exercises in which we use a pole, you may use your golf club, tennis racket, or even a broomstick. If you buy a weighted pole at a sporting goods store or use one at a gym, make sure it is no heavier than 5 pounds.

These exercises can be performed by those at any level and are incorporated into the specific sports programs found in the following chapters.

Biceps Curl Front (Strength)

- Stand in Pilates stance. Bring your arms directly in front of you at shoulder height with palms facing up.

- Inhale. Bend your elbows so that your arms are at a 90-degree angle, creating resistance with your biceps.

- Push the arms back out to straighten, again resisting the weights. Exhale.

- Repeat 5 to 10 times.

Tip: Keep your elbows at shoulder height while bending the elbow. You may add 5 repetitions to strengthen a weak arm.

Benefit for Sports: Scapular stability; control.

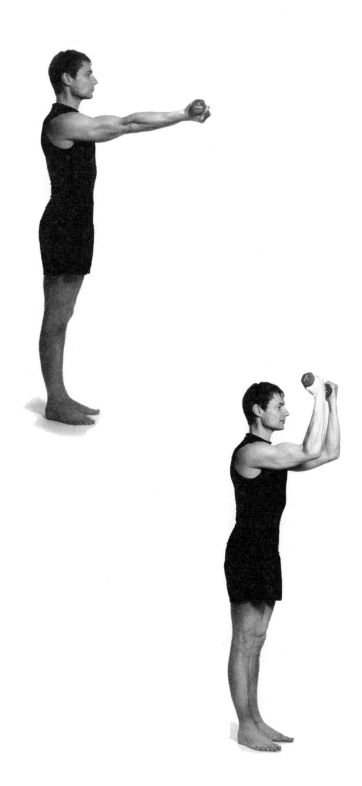

Side to Side (Mobility)

- Begin with your arms by your sides. Bend your right arm and bring it up the side of your body until it is raised straight. Keep your elbow close to your ear.

- Inhale. Lift the powerhouse and stretch over to the left side, making sure that you are lengthening your torso and not collapsing your right side.

- Bend your right elbow so your arm touches your left ear to increase the stretch.

- Straighten your arm. Lengthen the torso to return to center. Exhale.

- Bring your right arm down the side of your body and switch sides.

- Repeat 2 to 4 times each side.

Tip: Keep lifting both sides (not dropping or "crunching") of your waist while stretching to the side. If necessary you may add one more repetition for the tighter side and hold the stretch.

Benefit for Sports: Postural strength; flexibility for the sides.

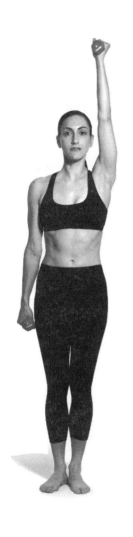

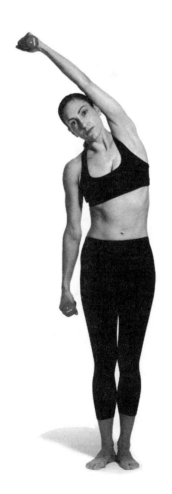

Zip Up (Strength/Control)

- Bring your weights together in front of your hips with your palms facing your legs.

- Inhale and bend your elbows out to the sides as you lift the weights straight up the center of your body all the way to your chin.

- Exhale and push the weights back down, using resistance with your muscles against the weights.

- Repeat 5 to 10 times.

Tip: Keep your elbows above your wrists and your shoulders down when in the up position. You may add 5 repetitions to strengthen a weak side.

Advanced Challenge: As you lift the weight, rise up to your toes (releve). Repeat 5 times with flat feet and 5 times on releve, keeping heels up the entire time.

Benefit for Sports: Scapular stability; balance; to strengthen the lower leg.

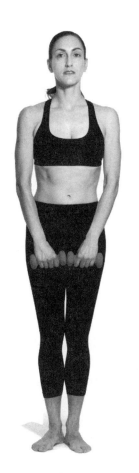
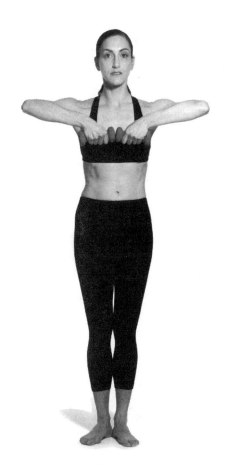

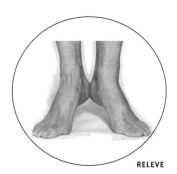

RELEVE

ʃhaving (Strength)

- Bring your arms in front of you and above your head. Bend your elbows to the sides with your hands/weights together at the base of your head.

- Inhale. Keep your elbows as wide as possible as you lift your arms up overhead, keeping the hands/weights together.

- Exhale. Bend your arms back down behind your head.

- Lift the arms again.

- Repeat 5 to 10 times.

Tip: Maintain one straight line from toes to fingers while lifting the arms. You may add 5 repetitions to strengthen a weak side.

Advanced Challenge: As you raise the weights, rise up to your toes (releve).

Benefit for Sports: Scapular stability; balance; to strengthen the lower leg.

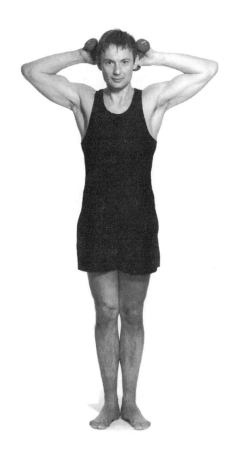

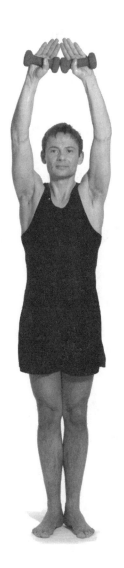

The Bug (Strength)

- Place your feet in a parallel position, hip distance apart. Bend your knees and bend your torso forward from the waist so that your back is flat.

- Let your arms hang down, keeping your elbows slightly bent.

- Inhale and open your arms out to the sides, pushing through the air, bringing your shoulder blades together.

- Exhale and pull the arms together back to center.

- Repeat 5 to 10 times.

Tip: Keep your powerhouse engaged as you lift your arms. You may add 5 repetitions to strengthen a weaker side.

Benefit for Sports: Scapular stability; postural strength.

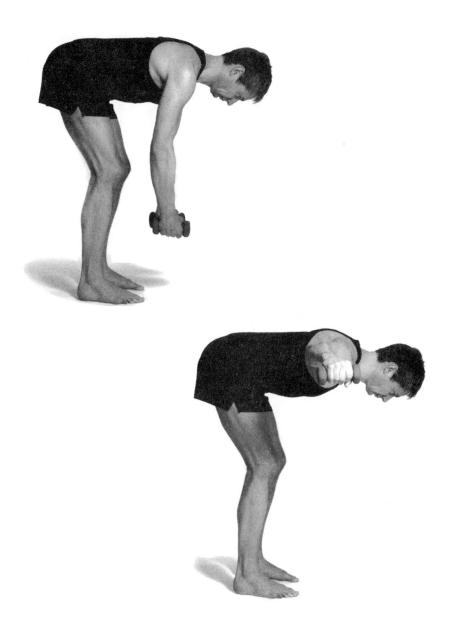

Chest Expansion (Mobility)

- Standing in Pilates stance, lift your arms straight in front of your body until they are shoulder level.

- Inhale. Pull your arms down close to your side and back behind your body. Draw your stomach in, bring your shoulder blades together, and open your chest.

- Holding the breath, look to the right side, then the left, and back to center.

- Exhale. Release the arms back to starting position.

- Repeat 2 times on each side.

Tip: Try to feel the shoulder blades coming together while pushing your chest out.

Advanced Challenge: As you pull the arms down, rise up to your toes (releve).

Benefit for Sports: Scapular stability; postural strength.

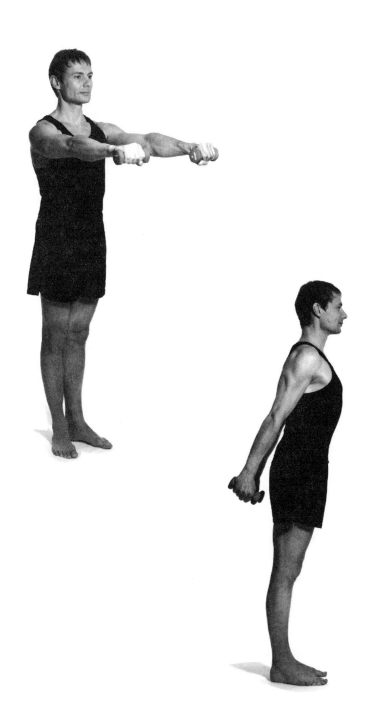

Low Curls (Strength)

- Place your feet in a parallel position, hip-distance apart. Bend your knees and bend your torso forward from the waist so that your back is flat.

- Inhale. Bend your elbows so they are pointing behind you close to your sides. Your hands should be close to your shoulders.

- Extend your arms back to straighten, squeezing them close to your sides.

- Bend your arms in, returning to home position. Exhale.

- Repeat 8 to 10 times.

Tip: Keep your stomach lifted to maintain a flat back. You may add 5 repetitions to strengthen a weaker side

Benefit for Sports: Postural strength; to strengthen biceps and triceps.

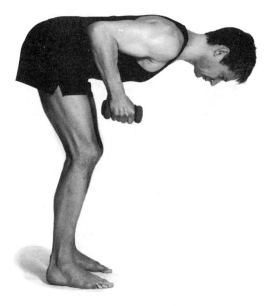

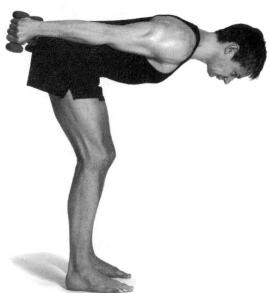

Wrist Raise (Strength)

- Stand with your feet in Pilates stance, holding a pole in your right hand close to the end.

- Keeping your elbow by your side and your palm turned in, lift the far end of the pole and lower the rear end without moving your arm. Use the strength of your forearm to raise the pole. Release slowly.

- Repeat 5 times with each arm.

Tip: Keep the elbow against your waist to support your arm.

Benefit for Sports: Prevent wrist injury; forearm strength for tennis and golf.

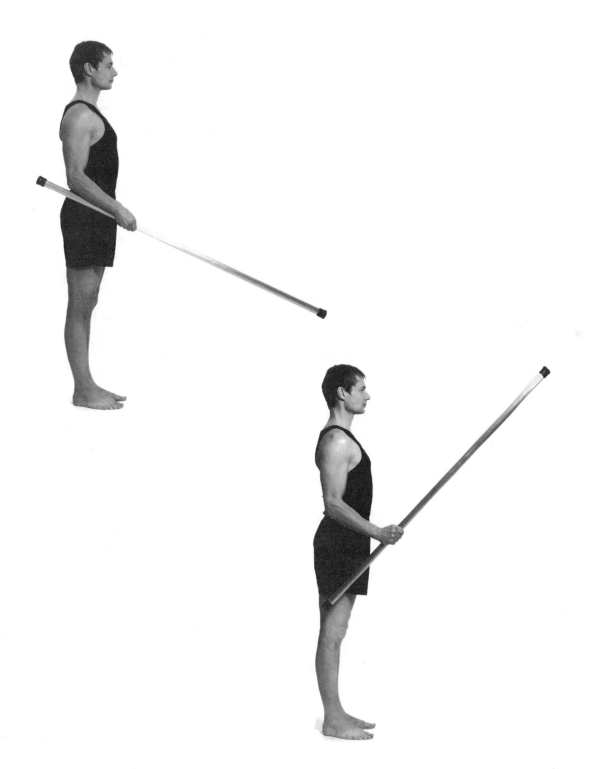

Wrist Supination/Pronation

(Strength)

- Stand in Pilates stance, holding the pole in the center with the right hand, with elbow pressed against your waist.

- With the right forearm at a right angle to your body and your palm facing down, rotate palm up and release your palm back down slowly.

- Repeat 5 times, then reverse by starting with your palm facing up, rotate down, and release slowly. Switch arms.

Tip: Keep your elbow against your waist to support your arm.

Benefit for Sports: Prevent wrist injury; forearm strength.

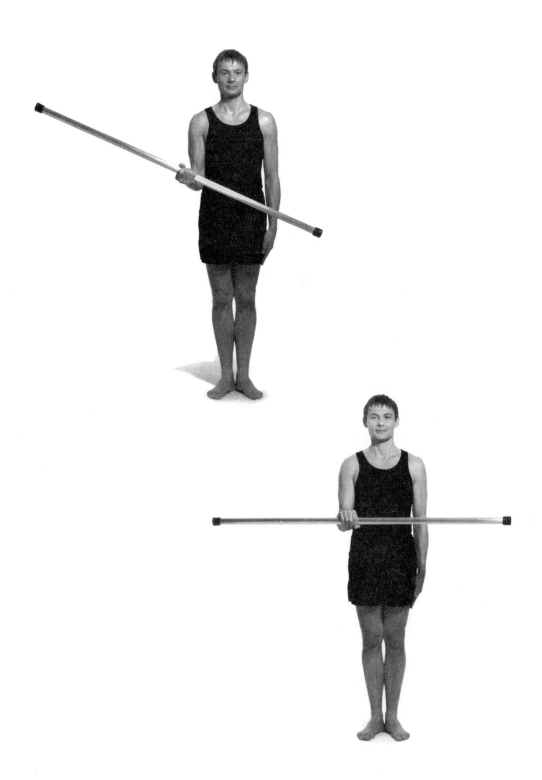

Wrist Rolls (Strength)

- Stand in Pilates stance. Grasp a pole in both hands with your palms facing down and raise it to shoulder height.

- Roll the pole forward, alternating between your right and left hands, 10 counts, articulating the wrist joints.

- Reverse the direction of the rolling for 10 counts.

Tip: Keep arms still as only the wrist is moving.

Advanced Challenge: Work your way up to rolling for 20, then 30 counts.

Benefit for Sports: Prevent wrist injury; forearm strength.

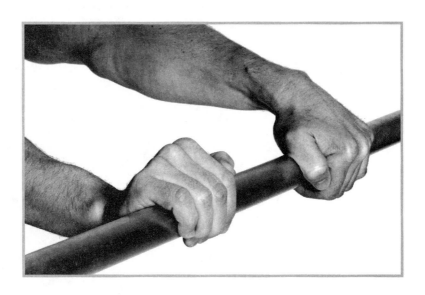

Ball Squeeze (Strength)

- Hold a small ball in one hand.

- Squeeze and hold for 10 counts. Release for 10 counts.

- Repeat 3 times. Switch to the other hand.

Tip: Try to feel the blood circulation in your hand as you release the ball. You may use a tennis ball or a soft rubber ball.

Benefit for Sports: Grip control for tennis, golf, cycling, and skiing.

6

Supplemental Exercises for Sports

These exercises were adapted from the Pilates apparatus to use specifically for the sport routines. They are advanced exercises and are incorporated in the sport programs to answer the individual needs and physical limitations of the athlete. You should not attempt these exercises before you have mastered the complete Pilates routine.

Footwork 1 (Strength)

- Lie down on your back with your hands behind your head and your shoulders slightly off the mat.

- Bring your knees into your chest, with your heels together and knees and toes apart.

- Straighten your legs so your feet are at eye level. Inhale.

- Bend the knees back into your chest. Exhale.

- Repeat 10 times.

Tip: Keep your stomach in while stretching your legs out in order to keep your lower back into the mat.

Benefit for Sports: Increase stamina; strengthen the powerhouse.

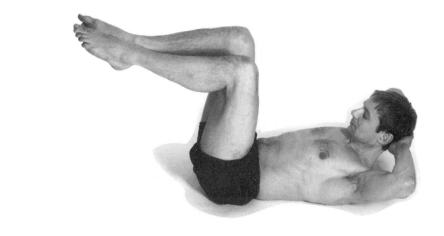

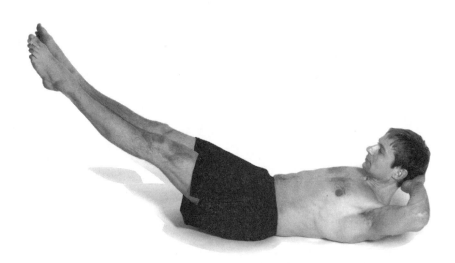

Footwork 2 (Strength)

- Lie down on your back with your hands behind your head and your shoulders slightly off the mat.

- Bring your knees into your chest, with your feet and knees together and toes gripped.

- Straighten your legs, keeping your feet at eye level. Inhale.

- Bend the knees back into your chest. Exhale.

- Repeat 10 times.

Tip: Keep your stomach in while stretching your legs out in order to keep your lower back into the mat.

Benefit for Sports: Increase stamina; strengthen the powerhouse.

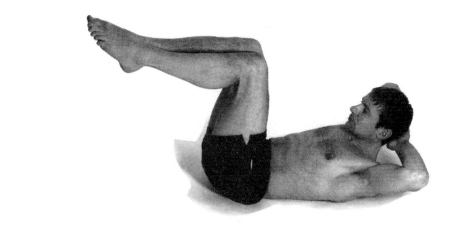

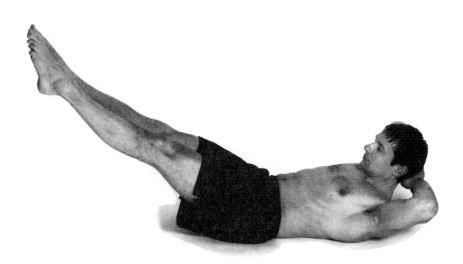

Rowing 3 (Mobility)

- Sitting up with your legs straight in front of you, bend your elbows and draw them back behind your torso. Your hands should be at chest level with your forearms parallel to the mat and your arms hugging your sides.

- Inhale. Bring your arms straight in front of you at a 45-degree angle.

- Exhale. Lower your arms in front of your body until the tips of your fingers touch the mat.

- Inhale. Lift the arms straight up next to your ears.

- Open your arms out to the side and press them down to the mat. During the movement, grow taller by lifting the stomach, engaging the buttocks, and lengthening the spine through the top of the head. When the arms reach the mat release the tension and exhale. Return to the starting position.

- Repeat 3 times.

Tip: Lengthen your spine by engaging your powerhouse when moving your arms up or down to sit as tall as possible. Keep your shoulder blades reaching down toward your hips.

Advanced Challenge: This exercise can be done with 2- to 3-pound weights.

Benefit for Sports: Stabilize scapula; correct postural alignment.

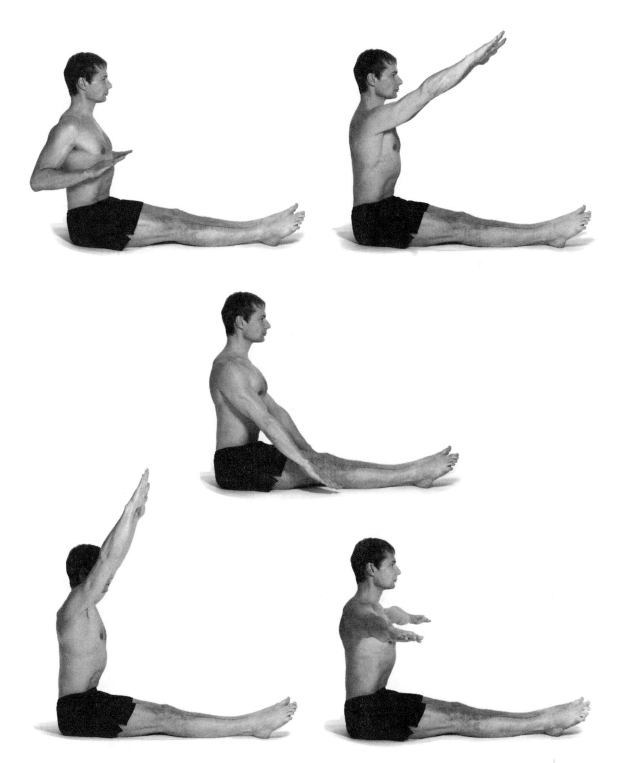

Rowing 4 (Mobility)

- Sit on the mat with your legs straight in front of you, feet flexed, and hands next to your hips against the mat.

- Inhale. Draw your stomach in and bring your chin to your chest. Roll down your spine to bring your head toward your knees. Stretch your arms forward, reaching for your toes.

- Using your powerhouse, begin to roll up to a sitting position. Raise your arms along with your body, keeping the shoulders relaxed as the arms reach upward. Exhale.

- Sitting up tall, continue to raise your arms up by your head. Inhale.

- Open your arms to the side and press them down to the mat, all the while lifting the powerhouse and growing taller through the top of your head. When your arms reach the mat release the tension. Exhale.

- Repeat 3 times.

Tip: Keep your shoulder blades down while lifting your arms above your head.

Advanced Challenge: Can be done with 2- to 3-pound weights

Benefit for Sports: Stabilize scapula; correct postural alignment.

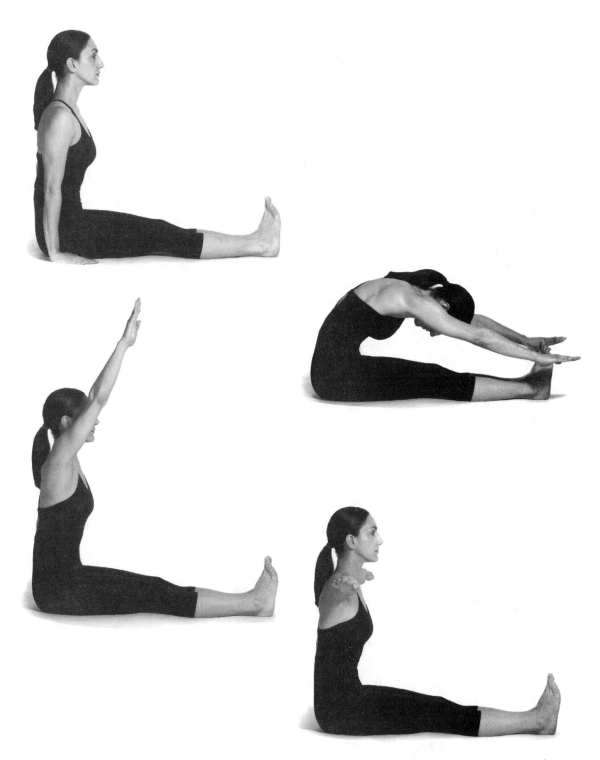

Pull Straps 1 (Strength)

- Lying face down on your stomach, extend your arms above your head a couple of inches off the mat.

- Inhale. Bend your elbows behind you and pull your arms to your sides. Straighten your arms as you reach your hands toward your toes, lifting your chest slightly off the mat while maintaining a long neck. Hold for 2 counts.

- Bend your elbows and return to the starting position. Exhale.

- Repeat 3 times.

Tip: Reach up and forward through the top of your head. Keep your toes on the mat.

Advanced Challenge: This exercise can be done with 2-pound weights.

Benefit for Sports: Shoulder strength; scapula stabilizer; improve shoulder range of motion.

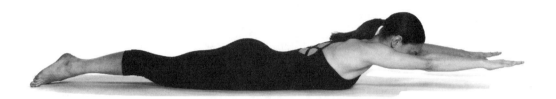

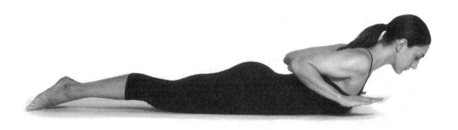

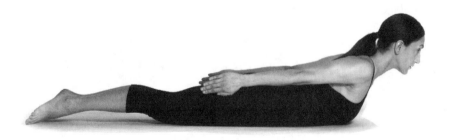

Pull Straps 2 (Strength)

- Lie on your stomach with your arms stretched out to the sides, hovering just above the floor.

- Inhale. Keeping your powerhouse lifted, pull your arms back to your sides, and open your chest, lifting your chest off the mat and bringing your shoulder blades together. Hold for 2 counts.

- Slowly go back to the starting position. Exhale.

- Repeat 3 times.

Tip: Reach up and forward through the top of your head. Keep your toes on the mat.

Advanced Challenge: This exercise can be done with 2-pound weights.

Benefit for Sports: Shoulder strength; scapula stabilizer; improve shoulder range of motion.

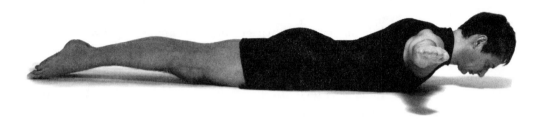

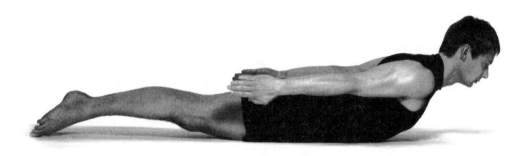

Teaser One Leg (Strength)

- Lie on your back with one leg bent and the other extended straight up at a 45-degree angle. Press your knees together and raise your arms above your head.

- Inhale. Bring your arms by your ears and roll up to a Teaser position, reaching your fingers for your toes. Hold for 5 counts.

- Roll back down, finding each vertebra on the mat by engaging your abdominal muscles. Exhale.

- Repeat 2 times each leg.

Tip: Keep your knees pressed together for stability.

Advanced Challenge: Add a twist after rolling up by reaching the arms in the opposite direction from the extended leg. Twist to the other side and roll down. You may add an extra repetition for a weak side when doing the twist.

Benefit for Sports: Balance and control; torso rotation for tennis and golf.

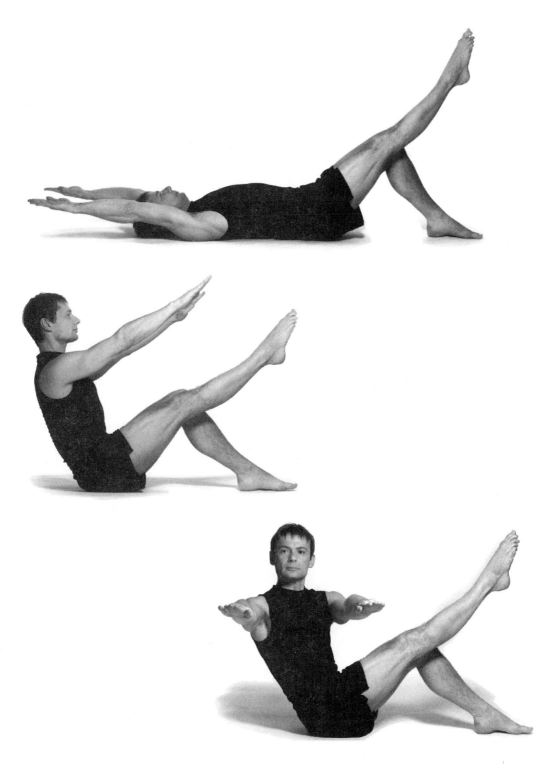

Thigh Stretch (Mobility/Control)

- Kneel on both knees, keeping them hip-distance apart. Raise your arms in front of your body at shoulder height.

- Inhale. Bring your chin to your chest and begin to lean your body back, maintaining a straight line from your shoulders to your knees.

- Using your powerhouse, bring your body back up in a straight line. Exhale.

- Repeat 3 times.

Tip: Keep your ribs in when returning to the upright position.

Advanced Challenge: Go even farther back and release the head. Bring your chin to your chest first, keeping your ribs and powerhouse in, and then bring the rest of the body up in one straight line.

Benefit for Sports: Loosen hips; regenerate tired legs, especially for tennis, running, skiing, and cycling.

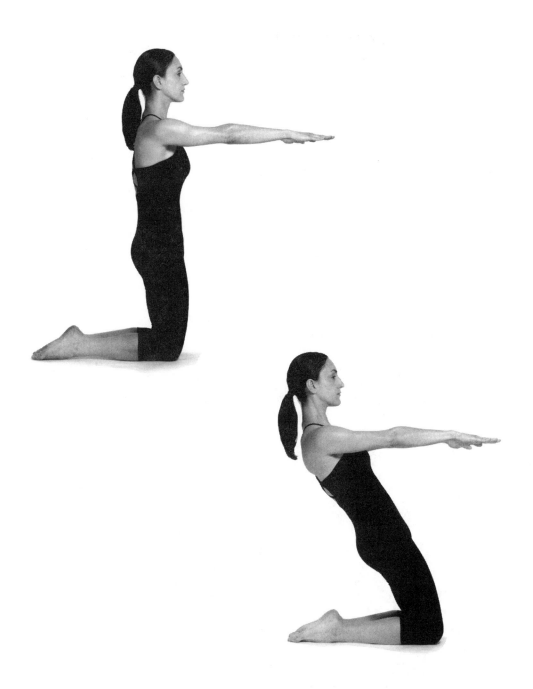

7

Exercises to Increase Power

Power is a combination of force and velocity. In many sports, power is synonymous with success. It is the way we measure ourselves against others. By increasing your power with the following exercises you can improve your game, your time, and your overall fitness. The exercises require a great deal of strength and control and are only done at the advanced level. They are incorporated into the sports programs that follow.

Knee to Chest (Control/Strength)

- Stand with your feet in Pilates stance and your arms crossed one on top of the other in front of your chest.

- Keeping your shoulders relaxed, inhale and raise one knee to reach your arms. Exhale as you lower the leg.

- Switch legs.

- Repeat 10 times each leg.

Tip: Try to step down on the same spot, with feet in continuous motion. Do not bend forward, but keep your upper body still while lifting your knee to the chest. For a more advanced workout, do 20 repetitions.

Benefit for Sports: Dynamic balance; coordination.

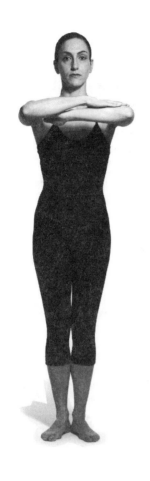

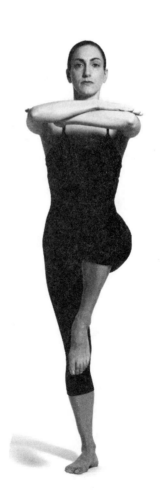

Knee to Side (Control/Strength)

- Stand with your arms stretched straight out to the sides and your feet in Pilates stance.

- Inhale and raise one knee to reach your outstretched arm.

- Exhale as you lower the leg.

- Switch legs.

- Repeat 10 times on each leg.

Tip: Keep your upper body still while lifting your knee to your arm by engaging the powerhouse, especially obliques. For a more advanced workout, do 20 repetitions.

Benefit for Sports: Dynamic balance; coordination.

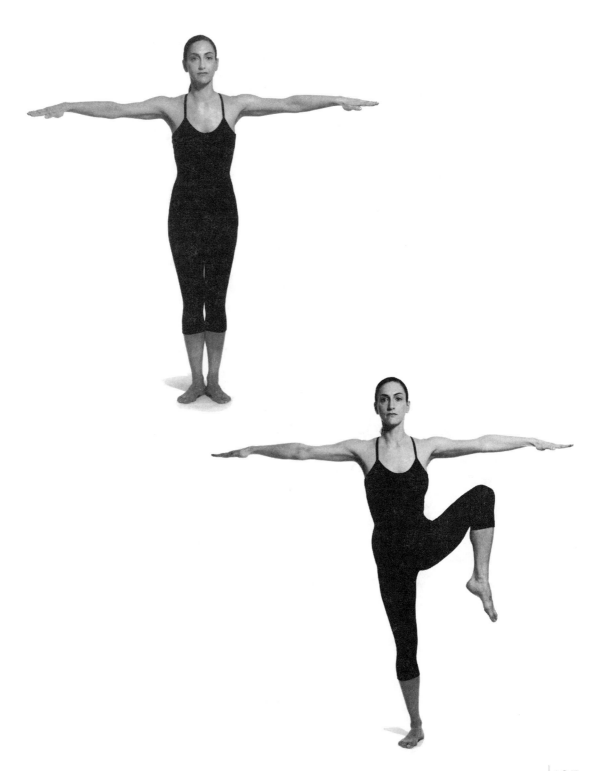

Lunges (Strength/Control)

- Stand with the heel of your right foot against the arch of your left foot and your arms by your sides. Your left foot should be slightly turned out.

- Inhale. Slide the right leg out in front of you and bend your right knee forward until it is at a 90-degree angle. Raise your arms to shoulder height in front of you and reach forward. Bend your torso forward, hovering above your right leg.

- Keep your hips even and use the powerhouse to slide your body back to home position. Exhale.

- Repeat 3 times with each leg.

Tip: Keep the weight of the body on the front leg. Make sure to keep your knee above your arch and not forward of your foot in order to protect the knee. You may also do this with 2- to 3-pound weights.

Benefit for Sports: Dynamic balance; muscular endurance.

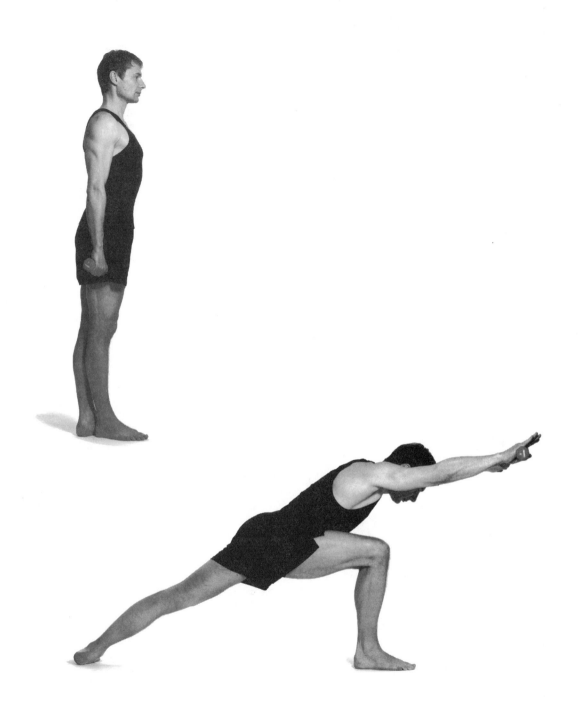

Jump Up (Power)

- Stand with your feet hip-distance apart and your arms stretched out in front of your shoulders.

- Bend your knees slightly and lower your arms to your sides, slightly away from your body, to prepare to jump.

- Inhale. Lift your arms to the ceiling as you jump straight into the air.

- Land with your feet parallel and knees slightly bent to absorb the impact. Land first on the balls of your feet and lower to your heels. Exhale.

- Repeat 5 times.

Tip: Can also be used as a cooldown exercise at the end of a workout by keeping the body relaxed while jumping.

Benefit for Sports: Increase power to lower extremity muscles.

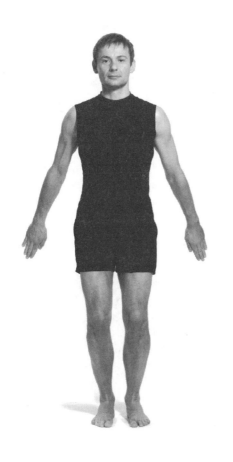
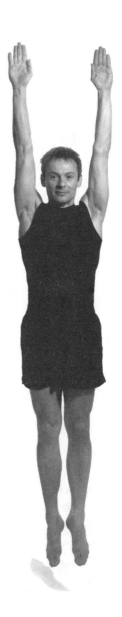

Jump Split (Power)

- Stand with your feet parallel and hip-distance apart and your arms by your sides.

- Bend your knees to prepare to jump.

- As you jump bring your legs and arms straight out to the sides, trying to touch your toes in midair.

- Land first on the balls of your feet and lower to your heels. Land with your feet parallel and knees bent to absorb the impact.

- Repeat 3 times.

Tip: Keep your focus on the muscular synergy while jumping.

Benefit for Sports: Increase power to lower extremity muscles, especially the outer thighs.

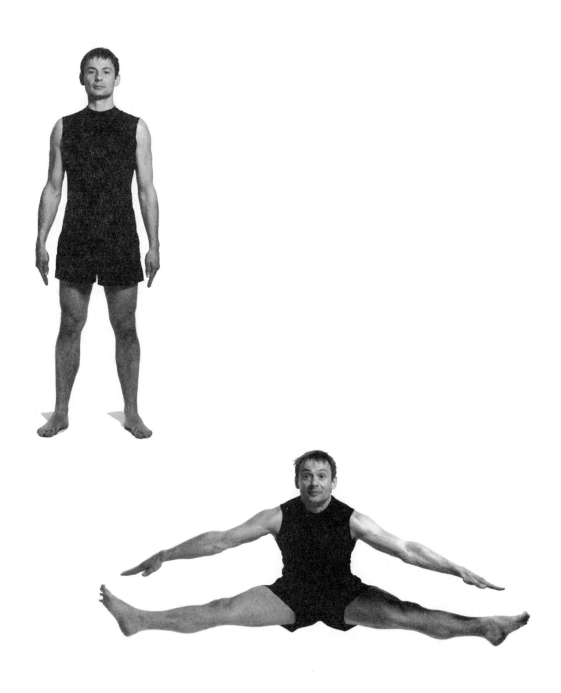

Stretches

Stretching is a vital component of a complete conditioning program. Since Pilates exercises already incorporate stretching with strengthening, a traditional warm-up is not necessary. For the athlete, the following stretches can reduce the risk of muscle and tendon injuries, reduce muscle soreness, enhance blood supply and tissue nourishment, increase flexibility and help you to cool down. These stretches are incorporated into the individual sport programs as well.

You may use a towel or an elastic exercise band in place of the pole if necessary.

Standing Swing with Pole (Mobility)

- Stand with your feet hip-distance apart holding a pole behind your lower back. Wrap your forearms under the pole so that it rests in the crook of your elbows.

- Slightly bend your knees. Twist your torso to the right and to the left.

- Inhale for 2 counts and exhale for 2 counts.

- Repeat 10 to 20 sets.

Tip: Keep your torso slightly bent forward, stomach in, and hips square while twisting the waist. Keep your lower back flat.

Benefit for Sports: Torso flexibility for golf swing and tennis serve, and swimming.

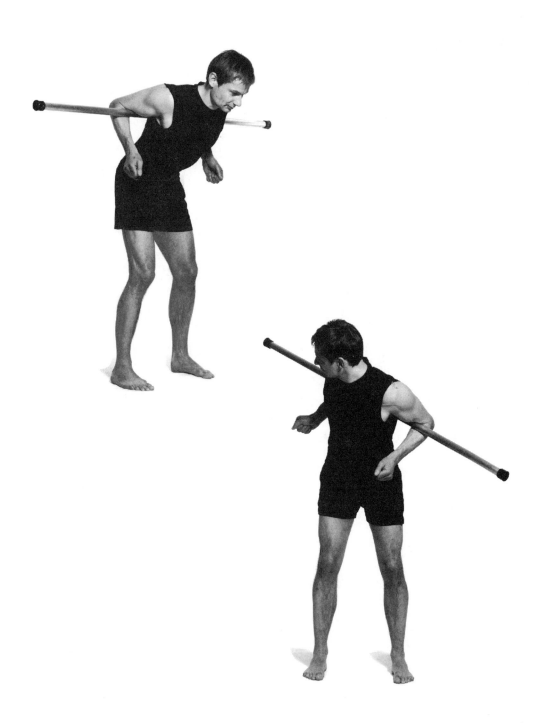

Stretch with Pole: Front/Back
(Mobility)

- Stand in Pilates stance holding the pole in front of your thighs, with your hands together.

- Lift the pole overhead and open the arms as wide as necessary to allow you to remain straight while reaching up and back.

- Reach your arms back, bringing the pole behind your back. Inhale.

- Lift your arms and come back to starting position. Exhale.

- Repeat 3 to 5 times.

Tip: Keep your powerhouse lifted so as not to arch your back. Keep your shoulders down.

Advanced Challenge: Reach for your toes with the pole as you come forward.

Benefit for Sports: Release tension in your upper back; prevent kyphosis for cyclists; shoulder flexibility for golf swing and tennis serve.

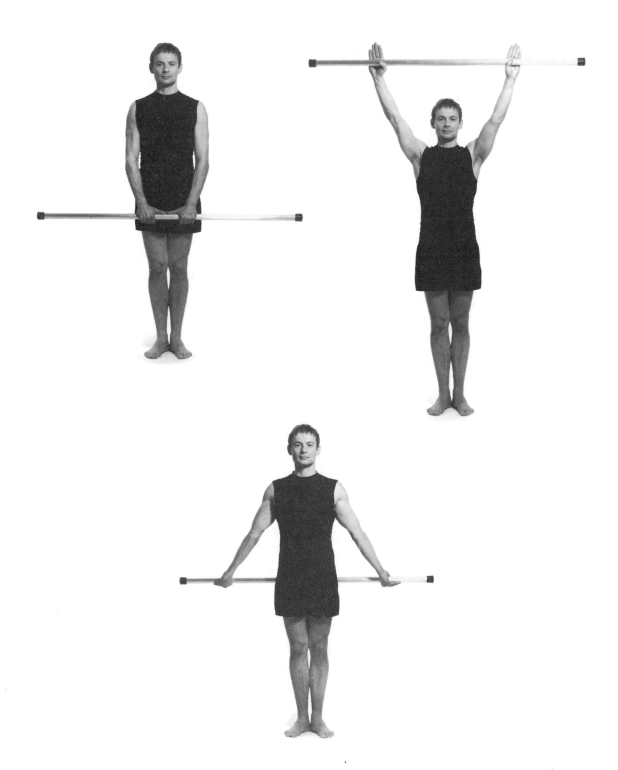

Side Down Side Up (Mobility)

- Holding a pole above and slightly in front of your head with your feet hip-distance apart, inhale and bend from the waist over to one side.

- Twist at the waist to face outward and roll down to stretch forward, reaching for the floor. Exhale.

- Twist at the waist again, moving through center to the opposite side. Straighten through your waist and come up the opposite side to standing.

- Reverse.

- Repeat 2 to 3 times.

Tip: Keep your hips square (facing forward) while twisting.

Modification: For sciatica, stretch only to the side, hold, then come back to center. Switch to the other side. Hold the stretch longer on the tight side.

Benefit for Sports: Improve torso rotation and hip and thigh flexibility for the golf swing.

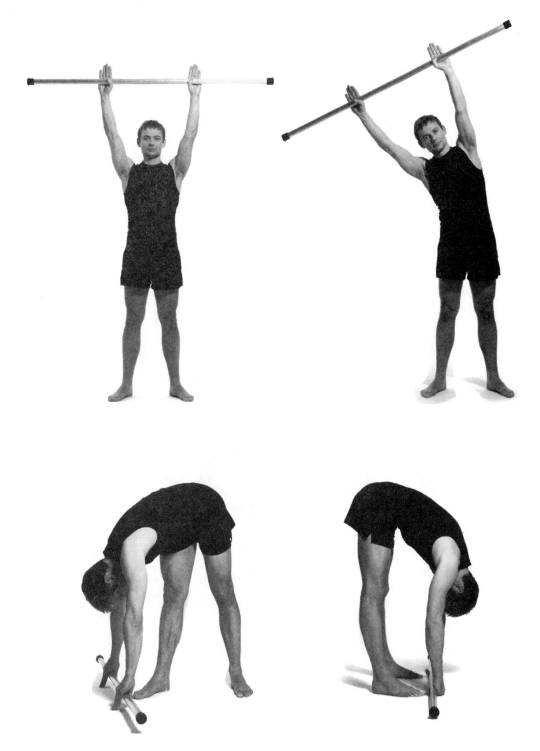

Stretch Leg Crossed Behind

(Mobility)

- Stand with your feet hip-distance apart. Lift your arms above your head, shoulder-width apart and cross your right leg behind the left. Inhale.

- Twist your torso to the left and then bend at the waist to reach the right ankle. Exhale.

- Hold for 20 seconds. Return to center. Switch sides.

- Repeat 1 time on each side.

Tip: Keep your legs straight and knees soft (slightly bent).

Benefit for Sports: Regenerate tired legs and improve leg flexibility, especially in the outer thigh and hamstrings.

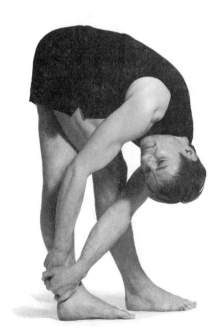

Calf Stretch (Mobility)

- Stand with your feet parallel and place your palms flat against a wall.

- Slightly bend your right knee, keeping the knee above your foot.

- Stretch your left leg behind you, far enough to keep your foot completely flat and pressed into the floor. Hold for 20 seconds.

- Switch legs.

Tip: Press the heel of the back leg into the floor to get a good stretch, and try to keep the upper body in line with the back leg.

Modification: The front leg can be raised and supported against a chair.

Benefit for Sports: Prevent ankle injury and regenerate tired legs.

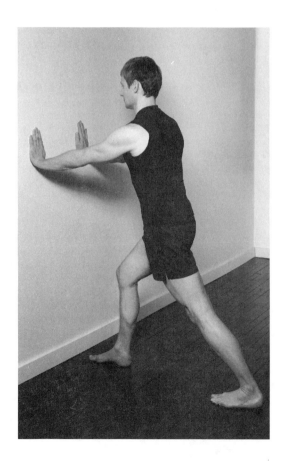

ʃpider (Mobility)

- Stand with feet in Pilates stance facing a wall. Place your palms flat against the wall, and stand far enough from the wall so that your arms are slightly bent.

- Engage your powerhouse. Inhale and begin to walk your fingers up the wall, as though you are typing, until your arms are fully extended.

- Continue the stretch by lifting your heels off the ground, and stand on the balls of your feet (releve), growing as tall as possible. Open your chest.

- Walk down the wall slowly. Exhale.

Tip: When your arms are completely extended, your shoulders should stay down, with the shoulder blades coming together. Make sure the body makes one straight line.

Benefit for Sports: Strengthen posture and correct kyphosis.

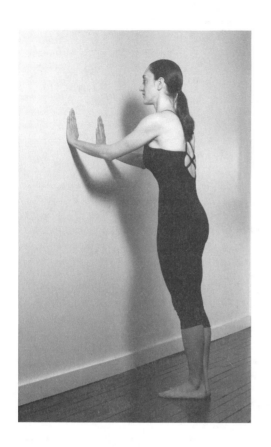

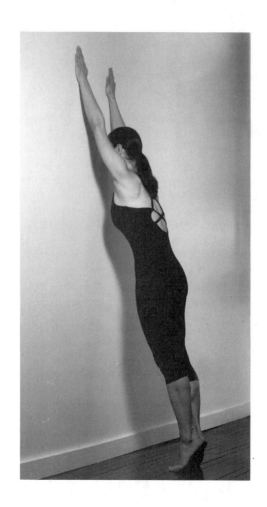

9

Cycling

Pilates builds power and develops correct posture, which benefits cyclists in many important ways. First, to boost performance, a cyclist must apply enough force to the bicycle and reduce external forces, such as wind resistance. In opposition to this, increased weight on the cyclist increases inertia, thus requiring a great amount of force to move the bicycle forward. Pilates will help cyclists create a lean, strong physique, increase endurance, and create a tremendous reserve of energy, things required for a long ride. Second, proper positioning on the bike is essential both for enhancing performance and preventing injury. Developing posture, balance, and control through Pilates exercises will help cyclists maintain a proper position on the bike, in turn helping them reach an optimal pedaling rate.

In this chapter, we will outline exercises to help cyclists achieve their athletic goals. As we explain the muscles and movements used while cycling, we will recommend specific Pilates exercises and routines in order to strengthen and stretch muscles as well as prevent injuries of the neck, thoracic spine, knees, lower back, and arms. At the end of the chapter, you will find two Pilates workouts for cyclists.

Correcting improper body alignment is key to improving performance. Cyclists need to work with exercises that will correct the constant curve of the spine, help them avoid deformation of the spine (kyphosis), and assuage pain surrounding the spine. Following are the primary fitness goals for cyclists that Pilates will address in order to promote proper alignment and enhance performance:

- Strengthen legs (quadriceps, hamstrings), calf muscles, buttocks, hip flexors, lower back, and abdominal muscles to improve effectiveness of the cycle stroke, which is responsible for propulsion of the bicycle.

- Build upper body strength to help the cyclist pull up on the handlebars and maintain posture and balance on the bike.

- Increase lower back and thigh (hamstring) flexibility to help establish the correct position of the trunk on the bike.

- Stretch hip flexors and quadriceps to avoid lower back pain.

- Correct muscle imbalances. Since cycling mainly works the quadriceps, it is important to work the hamstring muscles and to strengthen inner and outer thigh muscles to stabilize legs and keep the knee and hip joints in alignment. Also work to correct kyphosis (excessive flexion of the thoracic spine).

- Improve balance to minimize falls.

- Speed recovery of tired legs by using exercises that reverse gravity and facilitate blood return.

- Build better endurance through breathing exercises that purge your lungs of impurities.

Breakdown of the Cycling Stroke

There are many muscles utilized in the hips, knees, ankles, and torso during cycling (see Table 9-1). Also, the back muscles (erector spinae) and abdominal muscles (a balance between all four abdominal muscles) are working to hold trunk posture (flexion). There are two primary phases of the cycling stroke:

TABLE 9-1: MUSCLES USED IN THE PROPULSIVE PHASE OF THE CYCLING STROKE

MUSCLES USED	NAME OF MUSCLES	ACTION OF MUSCLES
Hip Joint		
Hip extensors	Gluteus maximus, hamstrings	Extension
Hip abductors	Tensor fascia lata	Lateral stabilizer, inward rotation
Hip adductors	Gracilis	Medial stabilizer
Knee Joint		
Knee extensor	Quadriceps	Extension
Knee flexor	Hamstrings	Flexion
Ankle Joint		
Plantar flexor	Gastrocnemius, soleus, tibialis posterior	Plantar flexion
Dorso flexor	Anterior tibialis	Dorsiflexion
Torso		
Torso flexors	Rectus abdominis, internal obliques, external obliques, transversus abdominis	Flexion
Torso extensors	Erector spinae	Extension

- *Propulsive phase:* The force provided by the leg muscles as the pedal is pushed down powers the bike forward. It is therefore necessary to have adequate strength in the calves, knee joints, thighs, and powerhouse.

- *Recovery phase:* As the leg circles down, the focus is to release pressure to the pedal, thus "resting" for the moment that the leg is down.

Although biking does not employ all of our muscles, Pilates works the body as a whole and will assure well-balanced development by restoring the balance between upper and lower body. Pilates can correct muscular imbalances, such as overloaded quadriceps, by stretching the tight hip flexor (iliopsoas) and the quadriceps and working the opposing hamstring muscles. In the table below you will find specific exercises for strengthening and stretching the muscles used while cycling, along with their specific benefit. These exercises are incorporated into the cycling workouts at the end of the chapter.

Injury Prevention with Pilates

There are three general categories of common injuries in cycling: (1) all-over body injuries due to a fall, (2) overuse injuries caused by undue stress to specific joints or muscle groups and (3) pain caused by improper posture on the bike, especially lower back pain when the bike isn't adjusted properly to your body. Below are some common overuse injuries for various parts of the body and tables of exercises for strengthening, stretching, and to help rehabilitate injuries.

Upper Extremity

Shoulder, wrist, and thumb injuries are common for cyclists. Shoulder and thumb injuries usually only occur when falling. Wrist injuries are common overuse injuries due to the pressure of the upper body on the palm of the hand.

EXERCISES FOR CYCLISTS

STRENGTHENING EXERCISES	STRETCHING EXERCISES
Rowing 3 to correct improper alignment	**Thigh Stretch** to speed up recovery of tired legs
Rowing 4 to correct improper alignment	
Pull Straps 2 to strengthen the upper body in order to pull up on the bicycle	**Spider** to improve posture and correct kyphosis
Twist 1 to increase postural strength and balance	**Stretch Leg Crossed Behind** to facilitate recovery and flexibility of the hamstrings
Jump Up to increase velocity for propulsion of bicycle	**Calf Stretch** to facilitate recovery of tired legs and increase flexibility
Neck Exercise to prevent neck trauma (or modified when neck is in rehabilitation)	**Stretch with Pole: Front/Back** to increase range of motion in shoulders for reducing kyphotic posture
Arm Weights	
Biceps Curl Front to control bicycle, strengthen upper body	
Low Curls to control bicycle, strengthen upper body	
The Bug to control bicycle, strengthen upper body	
Chest Expansion to control bicycle, strengthen upper body, and correct kyphosis	

Lower Extremities

Pain in and around the knee is the most common for cyclists, but foot and ankle injuries are rare. Cycling works mostly the quadriceps (front thigh) and can lead to a strength imbalance in the leg muscles, which could in turn lead to a muscle injury. It is necessary to ensure proper balance between quadriceps and hamstrings (opposing muscles).

Arms

Strengthening	Stretching

To control the bicycle and maintain posture when climbing hills:
 	
    Pull Straps 2 (p. 176)
 	
    Push-ups (p. 122)
 	
    Arm Weights: Biceps Curl Front (p. 144)
 	
    Arm Weights: Low Curls (p. 156)
 	
    Wrist Rolls (p. 162)
	Forearm extensor stretch—with the elbow straight and the forearm pronated (palm down), use the opposite hand to stretch the wrist downward.

Knee

Strengthening	Aiding Rehabilitation

To strengthen quadriceps and hamstrings and to correct misalignment of the knee through exercising the hip external rotator and lateral and medial stabilizer muscles of the knee:
 	
    Swimming (p. 101)
 	
    Shoulder Bridge (p. 70)
 	
    Leg Pull Down (p. 102)
 	
    Wall: Squat (p. 132)—paying attention to the amount of knee flexion
 	
    Jump Up (p. 190)
	Wall: Seated Leg Extension (p. 136)
	
	Wall: Standing Leg Flexion (p. 138)

Legs

Stretching the Hamstrings	Stretching the Quadriceps
Single Leg Circles (p. 30)	Single Leg Kick (p. 56)
Single Leg Stretch (p. 34)	Shoulder Stand Scissors (p. 66)
Single Straight Leg (p.38)	Shoulder Stand Bicycle (p. 68)
Spine Stretch Forward (p. 44)	Thigh Stretch (p. 180)
Side Kick: Front/Back (p. 72)	Rocking (p. 116)

Neck and Spine

Injuries are common in all regions of the spine (especially the cervical spine and lower back) due to the cycling posture. To prevent injuries from either overuse or impact, a cyclist should perform strengthening exercises for the torso, cervical musculature, lower extremity, and upper extremity muscles.

Neck

Strengthening	Stretching	Aiding Rehabilitation
To improve postural strength and decrease hyperextension of the neck: Wall: Neck Exercise (p. 140)	To improve cervial spine mobility: Neck Roll (p. 52)	Use your hands instead of the wall in the following exercise to rehabilitate the neck. Wall: Neck Exercise (p. 140)

Thoracic Spine

Strengthening and Stretching	
To reduce the kyphotic position:	
Rowing 3 (p. 170)	Rocking (p. 116)
Rowing 4 (p. 172)	Arm Weights: Chest Expansion (p. 134)
Saw (p. 50)	Arm Weights: The Bug (p. 152)
Pull Straps 2 (p. 176)	Spider (p. 204)
Swimming (p. 101)	Stretch with Pole: Front/Back (p. 198)

Lower Back and Pelvis

The lower back and pelvis is a platform that is responsible for powering the bicycle. Their stability will prevent misalignment when pedaling.

Lower Back and Pelvis

Strengthening	Stretching
The Hundred (p. 24)	Roll Up (p. 26)
Corkscrew (p. 48)	Single Leg Stretch (p. 34)
Swimming (p. 101)	Spine Stretch Forward (p. 44)

Routines for Cyclists

During the off-season, practice Workout 1 twice per week and Workout 2 once per week. During the season, practice Workout 1 and 2 once per week.

WORKOUT 1

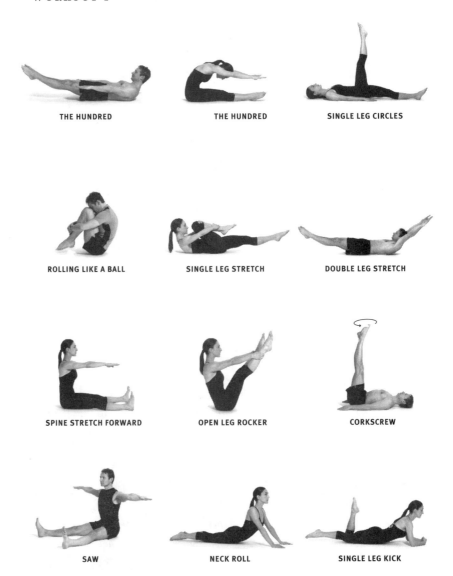

THE HUNDRED

THE HUNDRED

SINGLE LEG CIRCLES

ROLLING LIKE A BALL

SINGLE LEG STRETCH

DOUBLE LEG STRETCH

SPINE STRETCH FORWARD

OPEN LEG ROCKER

CORKSCREW

SAW

NECK ROLL

SINGLE LEG KICK

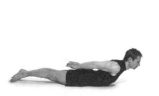

DOUBLE LEG KICK

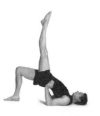

SHOULDER BRIDGE

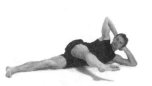

SIDE KICKS: FRONT/BACK

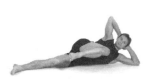

SIDE KICKS: BICYCLE

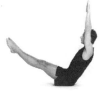

TEASER 3

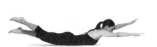

SWIMMING

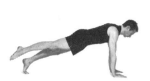

LEG PULL DOWN

THIGH STRETCH

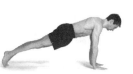

PUSH-UP

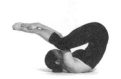

SEAL

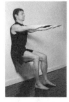

**WALL: SQUAT
(CAN BE DONE WITH 2-POUND WEIGHTS)**

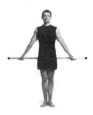

**STRETCH WITH POLE:
FRONT/BACK**

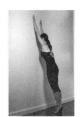

SPIDER

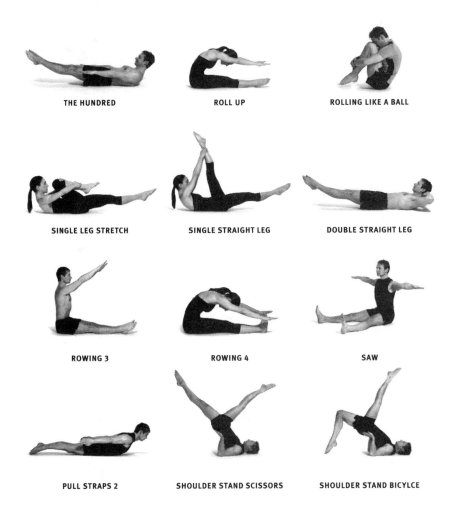

THE HUNDRED

ROLL UP

ROLLING LIKE A BALL

SINGLE LEG STRETCH

SINGLE STRAIGHT LEG

DOUBLE STRAIGHT LEG

ROWING 3

ROWING 4

SAW

PULL STRAPS 2

SHOULDER STAND SCISSORS

SHOULDER STAND BICYLCE

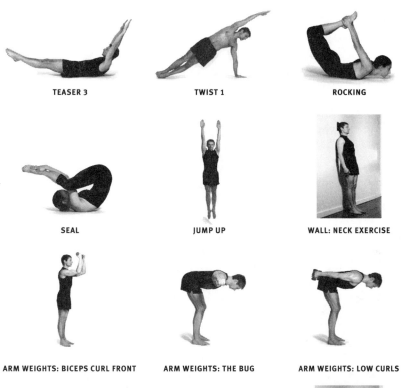

TEASER 3

TWIST 1

ROCKING

SEAL

JUMP UP

WALL: NECK EXERCISE

ARM WEIGHTS: BICEPS CURL FRONT

ARM WEIGHTS: THE BUG

ARM WEIGHTS: LOW CURLS

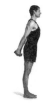

**ARM WEIGHTS:
CHEST EXPANSION**

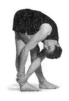

STRETCHED LEG CROSSED BEHIND

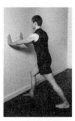

CALF STRETCH

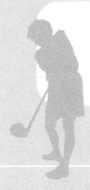

10

Golf

The Pilates method can be effectively used to better one's golf game by improving strength, endurance, muscle control (especially the core), and posture by strengthening different stabilizer muscles (such as the scapular stabilizers). The Pilates mind/body connection, learned from the six principles in Chapter 1, can help you achieve the concentration necessary to accomplish the stillness fundamental in golf. In this chapter, we will outline exercises to help golfers achieve their athletic goals. As we explain the muscles and movements used while golfing, we will recommend specific Pilates exercises and routines in order to strengthen and stretch muscles as well as prevent injuries of the shoulders (rotator cuff muscles) and of the lower back and knees, and correct muscular imbalances due to the one-sided nature of golf. At the end of the chapter, you will find two Pilates workouts for golfers. The ability to energetically play eighteen holes of golf requires the essential elements of a Pilates routine: coordination, balance, strength, endurance, flexibility, and mental stamina. You will find all of the exercises in the Pilates golf routine serve a specific purpose to improve your game and overall physique and prolong your golfing career:

- Strengthen the powerhouse because balance is necessary for a steady swing and will help stabilize the spine, which aids in injury prevention.

- Minimize risk of lower back injury, improve postural habits with lower back (lumbar spine) stabilizing exercises and strengthening abdominal exercises.

- Increase back of thighs (hamstrings) flexibility. Mobility and flexibility exercises should be incorporated with consideration for the setup position.

- Extend leg endurance by strengthening the legs in order to prevent fatigue.

- Improve torso rotation and shoulder and hip joint flexibility to create greater energy and momentum potential.

- Strengthen hand/wrist area, which transfers a great deal of energy from impact with the ball, by strengthening the whole arm from shoulder to hand.

- Correct muscle imbalances, which lead to injury. The weaker side will be exercised to overcome imbalances created by the golf game.

TABLE 10-1: MUSCLES USED IN THE GOLF SWING

MUSCLES USED	NAME OF MUSCLES	ACTION OF MUSCLES
Shoulder Joint		
Rotator cuff muscles	Teres major, infraspinatus, supraspinatus, subscapularis	External rotation, internal rotation, abduction, adduction
Shoulder adductors	Pectoralis major, latissimus dorsi, teres major	Adduction
Shoulder abductors	Middle deltoid, supraspinatus	Abduction
Scapula		
Scapula stabilizer muscles	Trapezius, rhomboids, levator scapulae	Scapula fixator
Torso		
Back extensor	Erector spinae	Extension
Torso rotators	Erector spinae, external obliques, internal oblques	Torso rotation
Torso flexors	Abdominals	Flexion
Hip Joint		
Hip extensor	Gluteus maximus, hamstrings	Extension
Hip rotators: External rotators	Gluteus maximus, gluteus medius, deep rotators, iliopsoas	Outward rotation
Hip rotators: Internal rotators	Gluteus medius, gluteus minimus, tensor fascia lata	Inward rotation
Knee Joint		
Knee flexor	Hamstrings	Flexion
Knee extensor	Quadriceps	Extension
Wrist		
Wrist flexors	Flexors	Flexion
Wrist extensors	Extensors	Extension

Breakdown of the Golf Swing

If we break down the main movements in golf, we can see how the body works while playing golf and how the specific Pilates routine for golfers can improve your game (see Table 10-1 for a list of muscles used in the golf swing). A great degree of rotation requires the golfer to have strength and control in the shoulder, upper back, arm, powerhouse, and lower back.

- *Setup:* the setup is the most important phase of the golf swing, as the quality of the outcome will be influenced by the setup position. Alignment, balance, and flexion are all key in this phase of the swing. A good setup position is important in order to avoid stress on the spine and to establish a proper position for the rest of the swing.

- *Back swing:* during the back swing rotation of the torso works in concert with the lifting and lowering of the arms.

- *Down swing:* proper rotation and shoulder stability is imperative during the down swing.

- *Follow through:* muscle activity diminishes as the swing is completed and held, which requires the golfer to maintain balance and posture.

Injury Prevention with Pilates

Poor posture and incorrect swing mechanics cause many golf injuries. For the upper body, it is imperative to maintain flexibility in the shoulders, good scapulothoracic stability, and prevent muscle imbalances. As for the lower body, it is equally important to keep range of motion in the hip joint, knee joint, and hamstring muscles flexible and to focus on overall leg endurance to promote better posture, balance, and to prevent fatigue. Below we have included specific exercises to address the needs of the golfer's physical condition.

Shoulder

The shoulder is a significant part of a strong golf swing. Accordingly, the shoulder muscles must be in good shape. Damage usually occurs in the lead shoulder (left shoulder in a right-handed golfer), which can

EXERCISES FOR GOLFERS

STRENGTHENING EXERCISES	STRETCHING EXERCISES
Rowing 3 and Rowing 4 to improve shoulder abduction/adduction for back swing, stabilize the scapula, correct shoulder alignment and upper body imbalance, and maintain proper posture	**Wall: Rolling Down** to release shoulder tension, improve posture, and correct lordosis
Pull Straps 2 to improve trunk stability, scapular stability, and shoulder range of motion	**Stretch with Pole: Front/Back** to increase shoulder flexibility and abdominal control
Teaser One Leg to enhance torso strength and maintain posture and follow through	**Stretch with Pole: Side Down Side Up** to increase torso and hip flexibility
Arm Weights	
Biceps Curl to improve scapular stability	
Side to Side to improve postural strength	
The Bug to improve postural strength and scapular stability	
Zip Up to improve postural strength and shoulder strength	
Wrist Rolls for hand/wrist injury prevention, and to strengthen forearms	
Wrist Supination/Pronation for hand/wrist injury prevention and to strengthen forearms	
Wrist Raises for hand/wrist injury prevention and to strengthen forearms	
Wall: Arm Circles to improve rotator cuff function	
Wall: Squat to prevent knee injury and improve postural strength	
Knee to Side to improve dynamic balance	

in turn cause shoulder damage and tendinitis. The Pilates program will improve the strength of the upper back and scapula stability and flexibility in the shoulders. Strength and flexibility are key in keeping the

SHOULDER

STRENGTHENING	STRETCHING
Rowing 3 (p. 170)	Roll Up (p. 26)
Rowing 4 (p. 172)	Rowing 3 (p. 170)
Pull Straps 2 (p. 176)	Rowing 4 (p. 172)
Push-ups (p. 122)	Wall: Arm Circles (p. 128)
Arm Weights: The Bug (p. 152)	Wall: Rolling Down (p. 130)
Arm Weights: Zip Up (p. 148)	Stretch with Pole: Front/Back (p. 198)

lead shoulder in good shape. You will find we have added specific exercises to compensate for a weak side due to lead shoulder complex.

ELBOWS, HANDS, AND WRISTS

Golfers elbow causes the elbow to be inflamed and can lead to degeneration of the area surrounding the elbow. A weaker shoulder also contributes to the development of tendinitis in the lead arm due to compensation with the elbow. If the shoulder is weak the elbow and arm have to work harder to compensate for this weakness, much like tennis elbow. Injuries to the hand and wrist are caused by the great degree of force used to connect with the ball. The elbow exercises listed below can be used to help prevent these injuries.

ELBOWS, HANDS, AND WRISTS

STRENGTHENING
Arm Weights: Biceps Curl Front (p. 144)
Modification: keep your elbows pressing into your sides.
Arm Weights: Wrist: Supination/Pronation (p. 160)
Arm Weights: Wrist Rolls (p. 162)
Arm Weights: Wrist Raise (p. 158)

Upper and Mid-back

Golfers occasionally have pain and hypomobility (loss of range of motion) in the upper and mid-back area from poor posture, which can reduce spinal rotation. Increasing tone and strength of the upper and mid-back will alleviate this pain and help golfers avoid back injury. In addition, appropriate stretching exercises will maintain good flexibility in the thoracic spine.

BACK

STRENGTHENING	STRETCHING
To increase tone and strength:	To increase mobility:
Rowing 3 (p. 170)	Roll Up (p. 26)
Rowing 4 (p. 172)	Spine Stretch Forward (p. 44)
Pull Straps 2 (p. 176)	Saw (p. 50)
Swimming (p. 101)	Spine Twist (p. 64)
Arm Weights: The Bug (p. 152)	Stretch with Pole: Side Down Side Up (p. 200)
	Standing Swing with Pole (p. 196)

Lower Back

Lower back pain is common in golfers due to dysfunctional movement (incorrect swing mechanics) and poor posture (poor stability in lumbopelvic area). Poor posture comes from lack of abdominal control and a lack of lumbar stabilization. Inflexibility of the hips can also lead to poor posture and lower back pain.

Knee

The knee is also stressed due to rotation and weight transfer while swinging the club. Balanced leg muscle strength is key to avoid injuries. We have developed a strength and flexibility program for the musculature surrounding the knee joint. We introduce specific exercises to facilitate recovery of knee injuries as soon as possible to minimize stiffness and loss of strength.

LOWER BACK

STRENGTHENING

To strengthen powerhouse and improve pelvic stability and posture:

The Hundred (p. 24)—modified

Roll Up (p. 26)—modified if necessary

Single Leg Circles (p. 30)

Single Leg Stretch (p. 34)

Double Leg Stretch (p. 36)

Single Straight Leg (p. 38)

Double Straight Leg (p. 40)

Criss Cross (p. 42)

Corkscrew (p. 48)

Teaser 1 (p. 90)

Teaser 3 (p. 94)

Standing Swing with Pole—modified (p. 196)

KNEE

STRENGTHENING	AIDING REHABILITATION
To strengthen the extensor and stabilizers of the knee: Side Kick: Front/Back (p. 72) Wall: Squat (p. 132) Seated Leg Extension (p. 136) Standing Leg Flexion (p. 140)	Wall: Seated Leg Extension (p. 136) Wall: Standing Leg Flexion (p. 140)

Neck

Injuries to the neck are uncommon, however golfers with a weak cervical spine can experience limited rotational mobility of the neck. Pilates movements can improve this impeded mobility and foster stability of the neck during the backswing.

NECK

STRETCHING
Neck Roll (p. 52)
Spine Twist (p. 64)

Routines for Golfers

Practice Pilates three times a week, doing Workout 1 twice a week and Workout 2 once per week.

WORKOUT 1

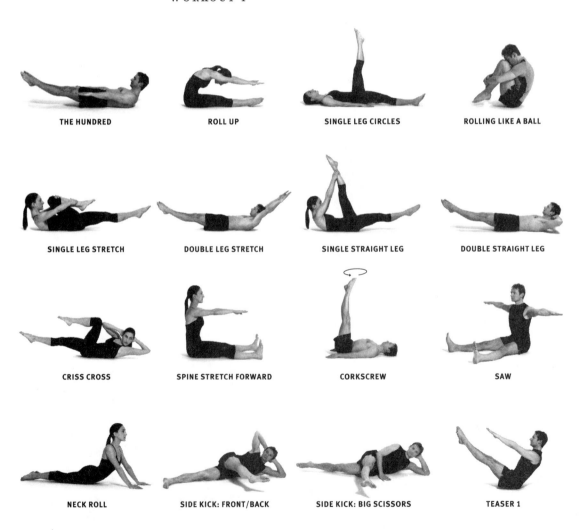

THE HUNDRED

ROLL UP

SINGLE LEG CIRCLES

ROLLING LIKE A BALL

SINGLE LEG STRETCH

DOUBLE LEG STRETCH

SINGLE STRAIGHT LEG

DOUBLE STRAIGHT LEG

CRISS CROSS

SPINE STRETCH FORWARD

CORKSCREW

SAW

NECK ROLL

SIDE KICK: FRONT/BACK

SIDE KICK: BIG SCISSORS

TEASER 1

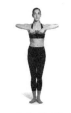

SEAL

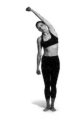

ARM WEIGHTS: BICEPS CURL FRONT

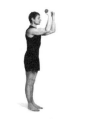

ARM WEIGHTS: SIDE TO SIDE

ARM WEIGHTS: THE BUG

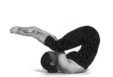

ARM WEIGHTS: ZIP UP

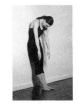

WRIST ROLLS

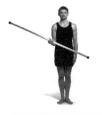

SUPINATION/PRONATION

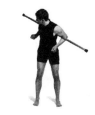

STANDING SWING WITH POLE

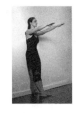

WALL: ARM CIRCLES

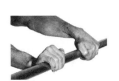

WALL: ROLLING DOWN

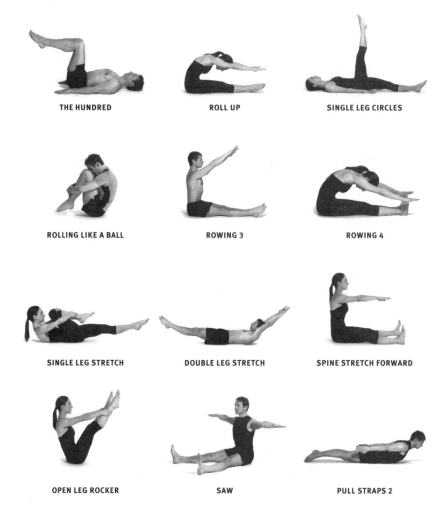

THE HUNDRED

ROLL UP

SINGLE LEG CIRCLES

ROLLING LIKE A BALL

ROWING 3

ROWING 4

SINGLE LEG STRETCH

DOUBLE LEG STRETCH

SPINE STRETCH FORWARD

OPEN LEG ROCKER

SAW

PULL STRAPS 2

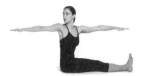

SPINE TWIST

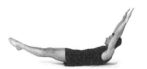

TEASER 3

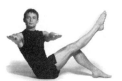

TEASER ONE LEG

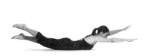

SWIMMING

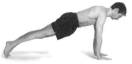

PUSH-UP

SEAL

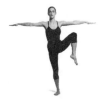

KNEE TO SIDE

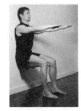

**WALL: SQUAT
(CAN BE DONE WITH 2-POUND WEIGHTS)**

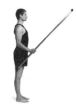

WRIST RAISES

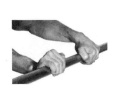

WRIST ROLLS

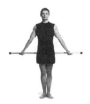

STRETCH WITH POLE: FRONT/BACK

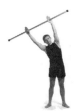

**STRETCH WITH POLE:
SIDE DOWN SIDE UP**

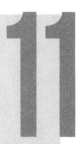

Running

One of the most important factors for runners is synchronization of breathing with movement. Joseph Pilates designed his method with the goal of improving the way a human body is nourished through breathing. When you breathe properly, you gain more stamina. Pilates believed in cleansing the lungs by rolling the spine. This theory was so compelling to him that he created many exercises that incorporate spinal massage by rolling. For example, Rolling Like a Ball stretches your spine, strengthens your core, and helps you to breathe deeply.

Pilates is also good for the runner because it includes stretching exercises for the hips, legs, and back. Too little flexibility can restrict movement. Pilates can be done to increase the range of motion with fluid movement. Moreover, runners want more flexibility without compromising their strength. In this chapter, we will outline exercises to help runners achieve their athletic goals. As we explain the muscles and movements used while running, we will recommend specific Pilates exercises and routines in order to strengthen and stretch muscles as well as prevent injuries of the knees, ankles, and lower back. At the end of the chapter, you will find two Pilates workouts for runners. The runner requires a balance of strength. A balanced pelvis supports the lumbar spine and sets the feet and legs in alignment. Combining all of these elements, Pilates can help the runner improve his performance and accomplish these fitness goals:

- Improve the overall physical condition and performance by strengthening the powerhouse.

- Stabilize the pelvis and give more range of motion and flexibility in the extremities (Pilates uses the trunk muscles to stabilize one segment, creating mobility in another part of the body).

- Stretch the hip flexor and hip extensor muscles. We get much of our power from our hips, thus the hip flexors are very strong and can create lordosis when they shorten.

- Help the injured runner who wants to stay fit by compensating for the absence of endorphins released by the body during running.

- Improve precision, posture, and alignment. Pilates develops a balanced body that helps you to keep your knees, ankles, hips, and hamstrings as injury-free as possible. The result of good posture for the runner is a balanced pelvis, as well as legs and feet in alignment, which is a very important part of the gait cycle. Any muscular imbalance will cause dysfunctional movement patterns throughout the body.

- Correct imbalances in the body. Lack of flexibility when running can cause a muscular imbalance. For example, a tight hamstring can stress your lower back by reducing anterior pelvic motion and making the thighs work harder at keeping the body properly aligned. Therefore flexibility is needed due to the excessive stress placed on the hamstrings during the gait cycle.

TABLE 11-1: MUSCLES USED IN RUNNING

MUSCLES USED	NAME OF MUSCLES	ACTION OF MUSCLES
Hip Joint		
Hip flexors	Iliopsoas, quadriceps (rectus femoris)	Flexion
Hip extensors	Gluteus maximus, hamstrings, quadratus lumborum	Extension
Hip abductors	Gluteus medius, gluteus minimus, tensor fascia lata	Abduction
Hip adductors	Adductors	Adduction
Hip internal rotators	Gluteus medius, gluteus minimus, tensor fascia lata	Inward rotation
Hip external rotators	Gluteus maximus, gluteus medius, piriformis, deep rotators	Outward rotation
Knee		
Knee flexors	Hamstrings: semimembranosus, semitendinosus, biceps femoris	Flexion
Knee extensors	Quadriceps: rectus femoris, vastus medialis, vastus lateralis, vastus intermedius	Extension
Ankle and Foot		
Plantar flexor	Gastrocnemius, soleus	Plantar flexion
Dorso flexor	Tibialis anterior	Dorsi flexion

Breakdown of the Running Gait Cycle

The running gait cycle represents the different phases of the limbs to produce forward motion. There are two phases of the Gait Cycle:

- *Support:* The runner is in single limb (leg) support.

- *Swing:* The foot leaves the ground and swings forward.

Several muscle groups are important in stabilizing the spine, foot, and ankle during running. The quadratus lumborum (torso muscle) stabilizes the pelvis while the opposite leg is pulled backward in running. The hip abductors and adductors stabilize the hip and pelvis. The knee flexors and extensors stabilize the knee, while the muscles of the ankle and foot stabilize the foot and restrain excessive mobility of the foot.

EXERCISES FOR RUNNERS

STRENGTHENING EXERCISES	STRETCHING EXERCISES
Footwork 1 to strengthen the powerhouse, to aid in the alignment of the legs, and to work stabilizer (adductor/abductor) muscles	**Lunges** to increase the power in the legs and dynamic balance
Footwork 2 to strengthen the powerhouse, to aid in the alignment of the legs, and to work stabilizer (adductor/abductor) muscles	**Knee to Chest** to increase power of legs and to promote hip flexibility
Thigh Stretch to speed up regeneration of tired legs	**Stretch Leg Crossed Behind** to stretch abductor (outer thigh) muscles and calf muscles to speed up recovery of tired legs
Arm Weights:	**Calf Stretch** to speed up regeneration of tired legs and to stretch lower leg muscles
Biceps Curl Front to help power yourself forward	
The Bug to stabilize the scapula and help keep the shoulders relaxed	
Zip Up to stabilize the scapula and help keep the shoulders relaxed	

Injury Prevention with Pilates

The Pilates method will help prevent running-related injuries through proper attention to alignment and balance. Pilates is a perfect form of rehabilitation due to the attention paid to the alignment of the hips, knees, and feet. By restoring muscle balance, a Pilates program will protect the joints and reduce strain on joint capsules and ligaments.

Runners, especially those who run long distance, have a high tolerance for pain. Many runners work through the pain and train regardless of whether their muscles are sore. But pain is a signal that should not be ignored. The result can be quitting permanently because of injuries that are not well healed.

Common injuries are caused from sources such as a rapid increase in mileage and hard or uneven surfaces including inclines, which can be responsible for knee and Achilles tendinitis. These injuries are most frequently seen when the body is tired or are caused by a lack of strength or flexibility. The repetitive nature of running often leads to mechanical stress resulting in overuse injury.

BACK

Poor posture can be caused by abdominal weakness, which may not allow you to support your spine properly and can cause back pain and have a negative effect on your breathing. Because Pilates exercises encourage a long spine, the tall upright stance gives your lungs space to function with efficiency.

Muscles that stabilize the back are found in the torso, or the core of the body (the powerhouse). Awareness and recruitment of these muscles will allow increased range of motion in extremity joints as well as prevention of trauma around the spine.

KNEES

Strengthening the muscles near the knees, especially the quadriceps, is necessary because of shock attenuation and the medial and lateral stabilizers of the knee. Due to a lack of power of the muscles surround-

STRENGTHENING	
The Hundred (p. 24)	Neck Pull (p. 60)
Roll Up (p. 26)	Jack Knife (p. 62)
Roll Over (p. 28)	Side Kick: Double Leg Lift (p. 80)
Single Leg Stretch (p. 34)	Side Kick: Big Scissors (p. 84)
Double Leg Stretch (p. 36)	Teasers 1–3 (pp. 90–94)
Single Straight Leg (p. 38)	Footwork 1 (p. 166)
Double Straight Leg (p. 40)	Footwork 2 (p. 168)
Criss Cross (p. 42)	

ing the knee joint, it is important to reduce the impact on foot contact. The stronger the surrounding muscles are, the more they will absorb shock and protect the knee.

KNEES

STRENGTHENING	STRETCHING
Swimming (p. 101)	Roll Up (p. 26)
Footwork 1 (p. 166)	Roll Over (p. 28)
Footwork 2 (p. 168)	Single Leg Circles (p. 30)
Wall: Squat (p. 132)	Single Leg Stretch (p. 34)
Knee to Chest (p. 184)	Double Leg Stretch (p. 36)
Lunges (p. 188)	Single Straight Leg (p. 38)
	Spine Stretch Forward (p. 44)
	Saw (p. 50)
	Single Leg Kick (p. 56)
	Shoulder Stand Scissors (p. 66)
	Side Kick: Front/Back (p. 72)
	Thigh Stretch (p. 180)

ACHILLES TENDON

The Achilles tendon is a frequent site of injury in the runner, especially when increasing uphill training, and also because of the hypovascularity (low blood flow) in the tendon. All Pilates exercises are designed to improve blood circulation in the body.

ACHILLES TENDON

STRENGTHENING	STRETCHING
To strength in the calf:	To increase flexibility, enhance blood supply, and nourish tissue in the calves:
Leg Pull Down (p. 102)	
Arm Weights: Zip Up (on releve) (p. 148)	Stretch Leg Crossed Behind (p. 202)
	Calf Stretch (p. 203)

Routines for Runners

Practice Pilates two days a week preseason and during the season, and three days a week off-season, with one day of rest between each workout. Follow Workout 1 twice and Workout 2 once per week.

WORKOUT 1

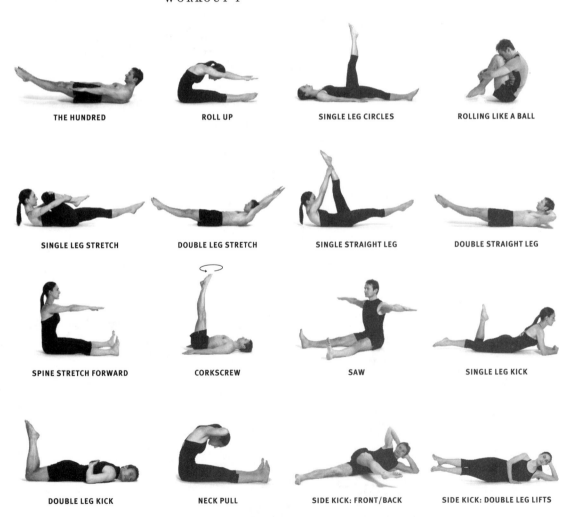

THE HUNDRED

ROLL UP

SINGLE LEG CIRCLES

ROLLING LIKE A BALL

SINGLE LEG STRETCH

DOUBLE LEG STRETCH

SINGLE STRAIGHT LEG

DOUBLE STRAIGHT LEG

SPINE STRETCH FORWARD

CORKSCREW

SAW

SINGLE LEG KICK

DOUBLE LEG KICK

NECK PULL

SIDE KICK: FRONT/BACK

SIDE KICK: DOUBLE LEG LIFTS

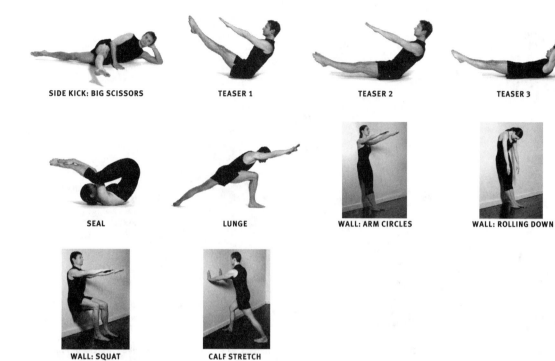

SIDE KICK: BIG SCISSORS

TEASER 1

TEASER 2

TEASER 3

SEAL

LUNGE

WALL: ARM CIRCLES

WALL: ROLLING DOWN

WALL: SQUAT
(CAN BE DONE WITH 2-POUND WEIGHTS)

CALF STRETCH

WORKOUT 2

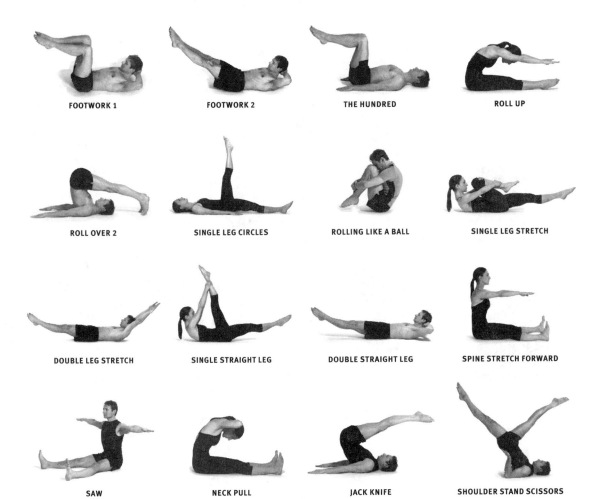

FOOTWORK 1

FOOTWORK 2

THE HUNDRED

ROLL UP

ROLL OVER 2

SINGLE LEG CIRCLES

ROLLING LIKE A BALL

SINGLE LEG STRETCH

DOUBLE LEG STRETCH

SINGLE STRAIGHT LEG

DOUBLE STRAIGHT LEG

SPINE STRETCH FORWARD

SAW

NECK PULL

JACK KNIFE

SHOULDER STAND SCISSORS

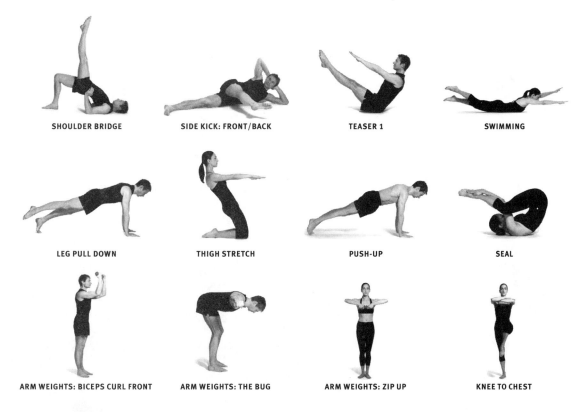

SHOULDER BRIDGE

SIDE KICK: FRONT/BACK

TEASER 1

SWIMMING

LEG PULL DOWN

THIGH STRETCH

PUSH-UP

SEAL

ARM WEIGHTS: BICEPS CURL FRONT

ARM WEIGHTS: THE BUG

ARM WEIGHTS: ZIP UP

KNEE TO CHEST

STRETCH LEG CROSSED BEHIND

12

Skiing

Skiing requires strength (especially leg strength to protect the knees), endurance (to avoid fatigue), and agility (to react to sudden changes in the terrain). Your body must be ready for the ever-changing demands of the weather and terrain. In this chapter, we will outline exercises to help skiers achieve their athletic goals. As we explain the muscles and movements used while skiing, we will recommend specific Pilates exercises and routines in order to strengthen and stretch muscles as well as prevent injuries of the knees, shoulders, lower back, and wrists. The Pilates Edge program for skiers provides two workouts that will get you down the slopes free of injury with exercises that combine strength, flexibility, and balance. Pilates will help you achieve these goals for skiing:

- Improve control and balance by strengthening the powerhouse to keep you upright and to keep you from falling.

- Strengthen the lower back and knee joints in order to diminish the likelihood of injury from the impact of falling, by strengthening the knee extensors and flexors and the powerhouse.

- Improve agility and decrease fatigue by stretching the leg muscles (calves), hip flexors (iliopsoas), backs and front of thighs (hamstrings and quadriceps), and lower back (back extensor, erector spinae).

- Increase power and endurance by strengthening the thighs (quadriceps and hamstrings) and buttocks (gluteal muscles) and the lateral and medial stabilizers (adductors and abductors).

- Strengthen the powerhouse (especially the obliques), which will help in making easy turns.

Breakdown of the Ski Turn

The fundamental skills in skiing are balance, rotary movements, edging movements (transferring body weight on the edge of the skis), and pressure control. Development of the powerhouse will help to keep your center moving squarely down the fall line. Both recreational and professional skiers use most of the lower body muscles and abdominal muscles while skiing and a large portion of the upper body muscles during pole planting (see Table 12-1 for a list of muscles used while skiing). Proper off-season conditioning of these muscles is required in preparation for skiing, which will also help to reduce skiers' injuries.

TABLE 12-1: MUSCLES USED IN THE SKI TURN

MUSCLES USED	NAME OF MUSCLES	ACTION OF MUSCLES
Torso		
Torso flexors	Rectus abdominis	Flexion
Torso rotators	Internal obliques, external obliques	Torso rotation
Torso extensors	Paraspinal muscles, quadratus lumborum	Extension
Hip Joint		
Hip extensors	Gluteal muscle	Extension
Hip abductors	Gluteus medius, gluteus minimus, tensor fascia lata	Abduction
Hip adductors	Adductors	Adduction
Knee Joint		
Knee flexor	Hamstrings	Flexion
Knee extensor	Quadriceps	Extension
Ankle		
Plantar flexor	Gastrocnemius, soleus	Flexion

The ski turn is divided into four phases:

- *Preparation phase.* A transfer of body weight occurs when the upper body shifts forward, requiring strength in the power-house, buttocks, and legs. A good starting position will impact the rest of the turn.

- *Turn initiation.* The skier initiates a turn by shifting the hips. Balance is required to make the turn without falling, in addition to adequate strength in the legs (quadriceps), lower back, and buttocks.

- *Fall line.* The skier increases pressure on the knees and hips, without compromising speed.

- *Turn completion.* The skier must maintain speed while preparing for the next turn.

STRENGTHENING EXERCISES	STRETCHING EXERCISES
Teaser: One Leg to increase trunk flexibility for turns	**Stretch Leg Crossed Behind** to facilitate recovery of tired legs and to increase hamstring and abductor flexibility
Pull Straps I to stabilize trunk (for correcting muscle imbalance due to lower body muscle overload) and to strengthen shoulders	**Calf Stretch** to facilitate recovery of tired legs and to increase flexibility of the lower legs
Thigh Stretch to help relieve overworked legs, to loosen hips, and also good for balance and control	
Twist 2 to stabilize trunk and increase flexibility of sides	
Wall:	
Squat to strengthen legs and improve balance	
Squat One Leg to strengthen legs, improve balance, and correct imbalances	
Knee to Chest to enhance balance for turns and to increase agility and flexibility	
Knee to Side to enhance balance for turns and to increase agility and flexibility	
Wrist Rolls to prevent wrist injury	
Jump Up to increase power of leg muscles	

Injury Prevention with Pilates

Skiing places great demands on the lower extremities and causes overuse injuries in the knees, as well as ligament sprains. Skier fatigue is also a factor for injuries, meaning the skier has prolonged contraction of lower back, leg, and abdominal muscles while skiing. Using the Pilates Method as supplemental training, you'll improve your sport and prepare yourself preseason in order to reduce skiing injuries that could keep you off the slopes.

Below you will find some common overuse injuries for key body parts and how to strengthen, stretch, and facilitate rehabilitation of already existing injuries.

Legs

The legs are obviously the most significant and overworked part of the body in skiing. For this reason it is important to strengthen the lower extremity muscles, especially the thighs. Many injuries occur when falling backward or from too much pressure on the knee joint when weight shifts forward from lack of strength in the powerhouse and poor balance.

LEGS

STRENGTHENING	STRETCHING	AIDING REHABILITATION
To strengthen muscles of the knee joint:	To speed muscle regeneration:	Wall: Standing Leg Flexion (p. 138)
Single Leg Kick (p. 156)	Single Leg Circles (p. 30)	Wall: Seated Leg Extension (p. 136)
Side Kick: Double Leg Lift (p. 180)	Single Leg Stretch (p. 34)	
Side Kick: Inner Thigh Lift (p. 181)	Double Leg Stretch (p. 36)	
Kneeling Side Kicks (p. 106)	Single Straight Leg (p. 38)	
Wall: Squat (p. 132)	Spine Stretch Forward (p. 44)	
Wall: Squat One Leg (if muscular imbalance) (p. 134)	Saw (p. 50)	
Lunges (p. 188)	Single Leg Kick (p. 156)	
Knee to Chest (p. 184)	Shoulder Stand Scissors (p. 66)	
Knee to Side (p. 186)	Thigh Stretch (p. 180)	
Jump Up (p. 190)		

Shoulders and Back

The shoulders and back are often injured by the impact when placing the poles into the snow or by falling on your outstretched arm. Newer extreme styles of skiing have emerged, using more jumps, turns, and aerial performances, which increase stress on the lower back. Below you will find exercises to strengthen the lower back, shoulders, and abdominal muscles.

SHOULDERS AND BACK

STRENGTHENING	STRETCHING
Pull Straps 1 (p. 174)	Roll Up (p. 24)
Swimming (p. 101)	Roll Over (p. 28)
Push-up (p. 122)	Double Leg Kick (p. 158)
Arm Weights: The Bug (p. 152)	Boomerang (p. 96)
Arm Weights: Zip Up (p. 148)	Wall: Arm Circles, with weights (p. 128)

HAND AND WRIST

Falling often causes hand and wrist strain. Strengthening exercises for the forearm and wrist will help to prevent injuries by improving strength in all the muscles surrounding the joint.

HAND AND WRIST

STRENGTHENING
Wrist Rolls (p. 162)

Routines for Skiers

Do three workouts per week, practicing Workout 1 twice per week and Workout 2 once per week. Preseason training should ideally begin eight weeks prior to going skiing.

WORKOUT 1

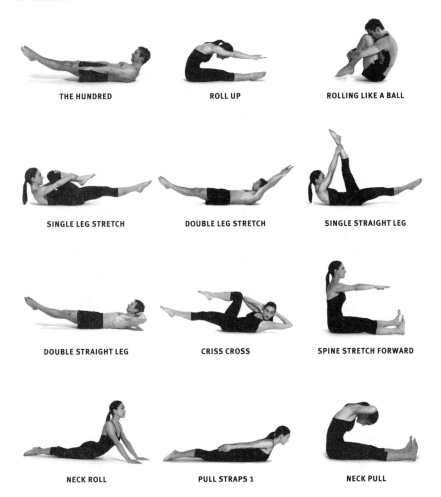

THE HUNDRED	ROLL UP	ROLLING LIKE A BALL
SINGLE LEG STRETCH	DOUBLE LEG STRETCH	SINGLE STRAIGHT LEG
DOUBLE STRAIGHT LEG	CRISS CROSS	SPINE STRETCH FORWARD
NECK ROLL	PULL STRAPS 1	NECK PULL

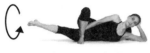 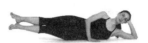 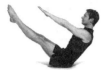

SIDE KICK: UP/DOWN   **SIDE KICK: DOUBLE LEG LIFTS**   **TEASER 1**

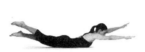 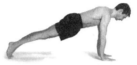

SWIMMING   **PUSH-UP**   **SEAL**

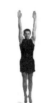 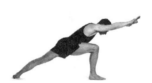

JUMP UP   **LUNGE**   **ARM WEIGHTS: THE BUG**

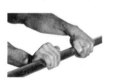 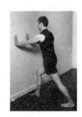

WRIST ROLLS   **STRETCH LEG CROSSED BEHIND**   **CALF STRETCH**

Workout 2

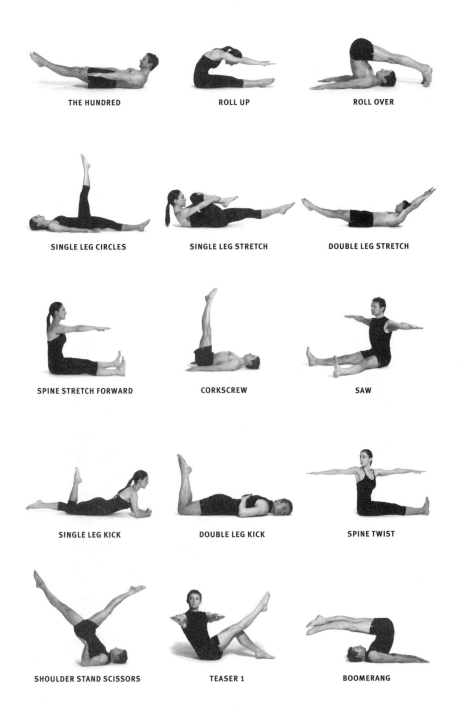

THE HUNDRED

ROLL UP

ROLL OVER

SINGLE LEG CIRCLES

SINGLE LEG STRETCH

DOUBLE LEG STRETCH

SPINE STRETCH FORWARD

CORKSCREW

SAW

SINGLE LEG KICK

DOUBLE LEG KICK

SPINE TWIST

SHOULDER STAND SCISSORS

TEASER 1

BOOMERANG

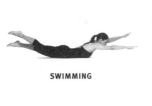

SWIMMING

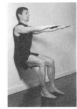

KNEELING SIDE KICKS

THIGH STRETCH

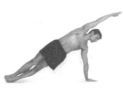

TWIST 1

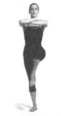

SEAL

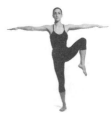

WALL: SQUAT
(CAN BE DONE WITH 2-POUND WEIGHTS)

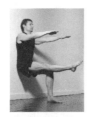

WALL: SQUAT ONE LEG

KNEE TO CHEST

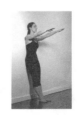

KNEE TO SIDE

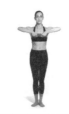

ARM WEIGHTS: ZIP UP

WALL: ARM CIRCLES

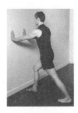

CALF STRETCH

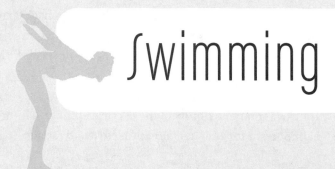

Swimming

13

Similar to Pilates, swimming is an all-body exercise, and most swimmers need a whole body—conditioning program to complement their pool exercises for maximum performance. Muscle bulk is not necessary to succeed in swimming, and the Pilates method will give you a toned and powerful body without building bulk, which will allow you to slice more easily through the water. Pilates lengthens the body and corrects bad posture, which will help maintain a horizontal position in the water. In this chapter, we will outline exercises to help swimmers achieve their athletic goals. As we explain the muscles and movements used while swimming, we will recommend specific Pilates exercises and routines in order to strengthen and stretch muscles as well as prevent injuries specifically of the shoulders and back. At the end of the chapter, you will find two Pilates workouts for swimmers. Pilates exercises are executed within the frame of the body, to help swimmers achieve their fitness goals, which follow.

- Improve flexibility in shoulder joints, lower back, and hamstrings for a better swim stroke. The lower back extensors shorten in swimmers because they must bring their head out of water for breathing, which creates hyperlordosis of the lumbar spine.

- Improve rotary flexibility of the cervical spine and hips, which is important for adequate breathing to avoid fatigue.

- Emphasize breathing exercises for regulative, rhythmic breathing.

- Promote balanced strength around the joints of the extremities and trunk. The underwater phase forces the muscles against a heavier resistance than when out of the water, which requires added strength.

- Strengthen the powerhouse, which will stabilize the trunk during propulsion through the water and helps to move your hips and legs when swimming. A strong powerhouse also creates a better balance: the more horizontal the body is positioned in the water, the less the form drag will be.

Table 13-1: Muscles Used in Swimming

Muscles Used	Name of Muscles	Action of Muscles
Shoulder and Scapula		
Shoulder extensor	Latissimus dorsi, teres major, posterior deltoid	Extension
Shoulder flexor	Pectoralis major	Flexion
Shoulder abductor	Anterior and middle deltoid	Abduction
Shoulder adductor	Latissimus dorsi, teres major, pectoralis major	Adduction
Shoulder internal rotator	Latissimus dorsi, teres major, anterior deltoid, subscapularis	Inward rotation
Shoulder external rotator	Posterior deltoid, teres major, infraspinatus	Outward rotation
Torso		
Torso rotator	Internal and external obliques	Torso rotation
Torso flexor	Internal obliques, external obliques, rectus abdominis	Flexion
Torso extensor	Paraspinal muscles	Extension
Elbow Joint		
Elbow flexor	Biceps	Flexion
Elbow extensor	Triceps	Extension
Wrist		
Wrist supinator	Supinator	Supination
pronator	Pronator	Pronation
flexor	Flexors	Flexion
extensor	Extensors	Extension

Table 13-2: Muscles Used in the Leg Kick

Muscles Used	Name of Muscles	Action of Muscles
Hip extensor	Gluteal muscles, hamstrings	Extension
Back extensor	Erector spinae	Extension
Knee flexor	Hamstrings and calves	Flexion
Knee extensor	Quadriceps	Extension

TABLE 13-3: MUSCLES USED IN THE BREASTSTROKE

MUSCLES USED	NAME OF MUSCLES	ACTION OF MUSCLES
Hip external rotator	Gluteal muscles (maximus and medius)	Outward rotation
Hip internal rotator	Gluteal muscles (minimus), tensor fascia lata	Inward rotation
Hip adductor	Adductor muscles	Adduction
Hip extensor	Hamstrings, gluteus maximus	Extension
Knee extensor	Quadriceps	Extension
Knee flexor	Calves	Flexion

TABLE 13-4: MUSCLES USED FOR RECOVERY

MUSCLES USED	NAME OF MUSCLES	ACTION OF MUSCLES
Knee flexors	Hamstrings, calves	Flexion

Breakdown of the Swimming Stroke

There are four different strokes in swimming:

- Free style

- Backstroke

- Butterfly

- Breaststroke

The free style and backstroke use arms in an asymmetrical reciprocal pattern, while the butterfly and breaststroke use arms in a symmetrical motion. Torso muscles are crucial for stabilization during propulsion of the torso through the water, and torso rotation depends on the coordinated contraction of all of the muscles in Table 13-1. The downbeat motion begins with forceful trunk and hip flexion, however, the abdominal muscles are the main driving force. During the upbeat motion, muscles contributing to trunk and hip are listed in Table 13-2.

There are three phases of the swim stroke, each of which utilizes different muscle groups:

- The *pull-through* is divided into hand entry, catch, power phase, and finish, and is the underwater portion of the arm stroke that creates forward propulsion.

- *Recovery* is the phase in which the reposition occurs. It is the out of the water portion of the stroke (see Table 13-4).

- The *leg kick* is the downbeat and upbeat motion of the legs.

Injury Prevention with Pilates

Creating a high level of performance and avoiding injury is only possible if there is a functional balance of the muscles that move the extremities and torso through the water. The most common injuries in

EXERCISES FOR SWIMMERS

STRENGTHENING EXERCISES	STRETCHING EXERCISES
Rowing 3 to prevent shoulder injury	**Stretch with Pole: Side Down Side Up** to increase flexibility in shoulders and hamstrings
Rowing 4 to prevent shoulder injury	
Pull Straps 1 to stabilize the scapula for greater pulling power	**Stretch with Pole: Front/Back** to promote shoulder flexibility and prevent kyphosis
Pull Straps 2 to stabilize the scapula for greater pulling power	
Jump Split to develop dynamic strength	
Jump Up to develop power in the lower body	
Arm Weights:	
Zip Up to increase scapular stability	
Shaving to increase scapular stability	
Wall:	
Squat to prevent back pain, correct lordosis, and improve postural strength	
Neck Exercise to prevent neck injury and correct poor posture	

swimming are overuse injuries, caused by overloading various muscles, joints, and ligaments. In order to avoid injury, the Pilates program will help you achieve better flexibility, strength, and control, thereby improving the form of your stroke.

SHOULDER

In the upper extremities, the shoulder is put through maximum range of motion during the swimming stroke, which causes micro trauma to the body. Because of the high physical demand on the shoulder (glenohumeral joint), a specific program of strengthening, stretching, and conditioning should be included three times a week during off-season.

SHOULDER

STRENGTHENING	STRETCHING
To stabilize and balance strength of shoulder muscle:	To increase flexibility:
Pull Straps 1 (p. 174)	Roll Up (p. 26)
Pull Straps 2 (p. 176)	Rowing 3 (p. 170)
Swimming (p. 101)	Rowing 4 (p. 172)
Leg Pull Down (p. 102)	Double Leg Stretch (p. 36)
Leg Pull Up (p. 104)	Boomerang (p. 96)
Push-up (p. 122)	Wall: Rolling Down (p. 130)
Arm Weights: Zip Up (p. 148)	Stretch with Pole: Front/Back (p. 198)
Arm Weights: Shaving (p. 150)	

NECK AND BACK

The neck and back are common injury sites caused most often by repetitive stress during turns and poor head and body positioning in the water. Back-injury prevention can be achieved by strengthening the powerhouse (especially the abdominals) because of the imbalance of strength in the trunk musculature in traditional swimming training, which emphasizes work of the trunk extensors.

NECK AND BACK	CERVICAL SPINE
STRENGTHENING	**STRENGTHENING**
The Hundred (p. 24)	Neck Roll (p. 52)
Roll Up (p. 26)	Swan (p. 54)
Single Leg Stretch (p. 34)	Snake (p. 110)
Double Leg Stretch (p. 36)	Wall: Neck Exercise (p. 140)
Single Straight Leg (p. 38)	
Double Straight Leg (p. 40)	
Neck Pull (p. 60)	
Teaser 1 (p. 90)	

LOWER EXTREMITIES

For the lower extremities, the knee is the most common injury site, especially during the breaststroke, due to the stress on the ligaments around the knee joints. It is imperative to keep the knee in alignment with the hip, which can be done by working into the joints and controlling the range of motion. To avoid injury *strengthen* the area surrounding the knee.

LOWER EXTREMETIES

STRENGTHENING	STRETCHING
To strengthen the area surrounding the knee:	To increase flexibility of hamstrings, back extensors, and hip flexors:
Single Leg Kick (p. 56)	Roll Up (p. 26)
Side Kick: Front/Back (p. 72)	Rolling Like a Ball (p. 32)
Wall: Squat (p. 132)	Single Leg Stretch (p. 34)
Jump Up (p. 190)	Double Leg Stretch (p. 36)
	Single Straight Leg (p. 38)
	Spine Stretch Forward (p. 44)
	Side Kick: Front/Back (p. 72)
	Stretch with Pole: Side Down Side Up (p. 200)

Routines for Swimmers

Swimmers should follow Workout 1 two times per week and Workout 2 one time per week off-season. During the season, do each workout once a week.

WORKOUT 1

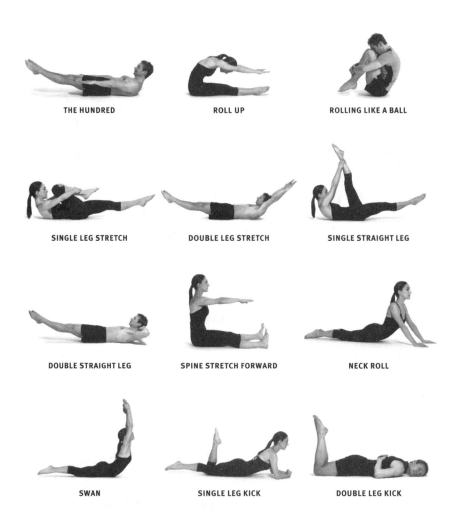

THE HUNDRED

ROLL UP

ROLLING LIKE A BALL

SINGLE LEG STRETCH

DOUBLE LEG STRETCH

SINGLE STRAIGHT LEG

DOUBLE STRAIGHT LEG

SPINE STRETCH FORWARD

NECK ROLL

SWAN

SINGLE LEG KICK

DOUBLE LEG KICK

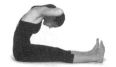

NECK PULL

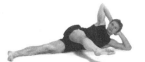

SIDE KICK: FRONT/BACK

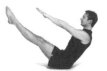

TEASER 1

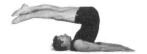

BOOMERANG

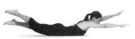

SWIMMING

SEAL

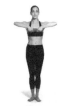

ARM WEIGHTS: ZIP UP

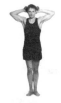

ARM WEIGHTS: SHAVING

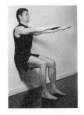

WALL: SQUAT

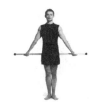

STRETCH WITH POLE: FRONT/BACK

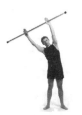

**STRETCH WITH POLE:
SIDE DOWN SIDE UP**

WORKOUT 2

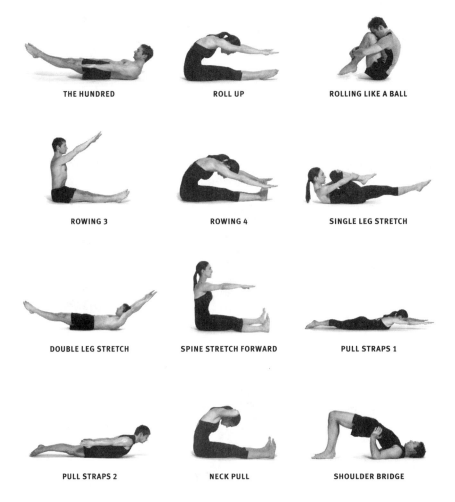

THE HUNDRED

ROLL UP

ROLLING LIKE A BALL

ROWING 3

ROWING 4

SINGLE LEG STRETCH

DOUBLE LEG STRETCH

SPINE STRETCH FORWARD

PULL STRAPS 1

PULL STRAPS 2

NECK PULL

SHOULDER BRIDGE

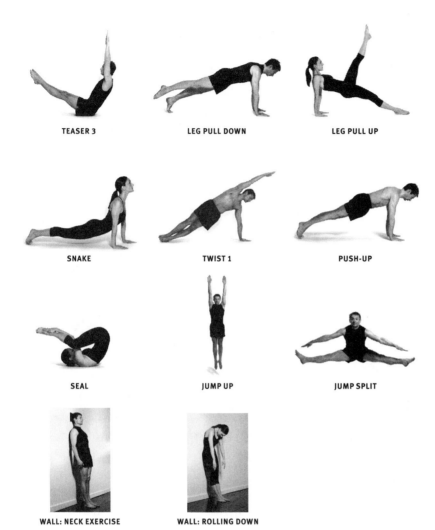

TEASER 3

LEG PULL DOWN

LEG PULL UP

SNAKE

TWIST 1

PUSH-UP

SEAL

JUMP UP

JUMP SPLIT

WALL: NECK EXERCISE

WALL: ROLLING DOWN

14

Tennis

In choosing a Pilates program for tennis players, we considered the dynamic nature of the sport, including the range of motion the body must achieve and the type of muscle contractions that occur during the sport. The fitness demands of the tennis player are quite high and require the players to have flexibility, strength and endurance, power, agility, and speed, combined with maintaining proper balance. When playing tennis, you must fully extend your arm over your head to connect with the ball. This kind of extreme range of motion requires considerable flexibility. A great deal of power is required to produce a strong serve. Additionally, a tennis match can last hours, during which time you are constantly running and hitting the ball. Each time you hit the ball, you contract your abdominal muscles, so you need good muscular endurance. The conditioning program in the Pilates Edge provides tennis players with a specific training routine to improve their overall fitness and performance but will also help to prevent injury.

In this chapter, we will outline exercises to help tennis players achieve their athletic goals. As we explain the muscles and movements used while playing tennis, we will recommend specific Pilates exercises and routines in order to strengthen and stretch muscles as well as prevent injuries specifically of the shoulders, lower back, and elbows. At the end of the chapter, you will find two Pilates workouts for tennis players. Following are the goals the Pilates Edge program will help tennis players achieve:

· Improve power of your stroke by developing strength in the powerhouse.

· Improve serve velocity by strengthening shoulders and arms.

· Increase flexibility. Poor flexibility of the key muscles groups (shoulders, hips) effects the proper execution of the strokes and often leads to injury. Having good flexibility will also help to reach the wide shots.

· Improve balance, as it is very important to maintain your center of gravity when changing direction. Good balance will allow you to be in the correct position to hit the ball.

· Improve lower body power to reach the ball as quickly as possible. Improve the upper body power to hit the ball hard throughout the match.

· Extend endurance, which will improve the ability to take in, transport, and use oxygen. Better endurance will prepare you for the quick transitions in tennis, in addition to keeping you in the game without tiring.

- Correct muscle imbalances that cause faulty movement patterns and may lead to joint strain and inflammation (tendinitis). The weaker side will be exercised to overcome imbalances created by the sport.

TABLE 14-1: MUSCLES USED IN THE FOREHAND STROKE

MUSCLES USED	NAME OF MUSCLES	ACTION OF MUSCLES
Shoulder Joint and Scapula		
Shoulder internal rotators	Latissimus dorsi, teres major, pectoralis major, anterior deltoid, subscapularis	Inward rotation
Scapula		
Scapula abductor	Serratus anterior	Abduction
Torso		
Torso rotators	Internal obliques, external obliques	Torso rotation
Back extensors	Erector spinae	Extension
Elbow		
Elbow flexors	Biceps	Flexion
Hip Joint		
Hip extensors	Gluteal muscles	Extension
Knee Joint		
Knee extensor	Quadriceps	Extension
Ankle and Foot		
Plantar flexor	Calves, gastrocnemius, soleus	Flexion

TABLE 14-2: MUSCLES USED IN THE ONE-HANDED BACKSTROKE*

MUSCLES USED	NAME OF MUSCLES	ACTION OF MUSCLES
Shoulder Joint and Scapula		
Scapula stabilizers	Rhomboids, trapezius, serratus anterior	Scapula fixator
Shoulder abductors	Middle deltoid	Abduction
Shoulder external rotators	Posterior deltoid, teres minor, infrapinatus	Outward rotation
Elbow Joint		
Elbow extensors	Triceps	Extension
Hip Joint		
Hip extensors	Gluteal muscles	Extension
Knee Joint		
Knee extensor	Quadriceps	Extension
Torso		
Torso Rotators	Internal obliques, external obliques	Torso rotation
Back extensors	Erector spinae	Extension

*The two-handed backstroke uses a combination of the muscles used in the forehand and one-handed backstroke.

TABLE 14-3: MUSCLES USED FOR THE TENNIS SERVE

MUSCLES USED	NAME OF MUSCLES	ACTION OF MUSCLES
Torso		
Torso rotators	Internal obliques, external obliques	Torso rotation
Hip and Knee Joints		
Hip extensors	Gluteals	Extension
Hip external rotators	Gluteus medius	Outward rotation
Hip internal rotators	Gluteus minimus Tensor fascia lata	Inward rotation
Knee extensors	Quadriceps	Extension
Shoulder Joint		
Shoulder internal rotators	Latissimus dorsi, teres major, pectoralis major, anterior deltoid	Inward rotation
Elbow		
Elbow extensor	Triceps	Extension
Wrist		
Wrist pronators	Pronators	Pronation

Breakdown of Tennis Serve and Strokes

During all ground strokes and the serve, the goal of the lower extremities and torso is to transfer energy to the racket. There are four phases of the tennis serve:

1. *Wind up*—the back, hip and trunk rotate, shoulder and elbow extend.

2. *Cocking*—shoulder and scapula stabilizers are active.

3. *Acceleration*—torso muscles contract, arm prepares for ball contact.

4. *Follow through*—after ball contact, arm continues forward motion.

EXERCISES FOR TENNIS PLAYERS

STRENGTHENING EXERCISES	STRETCHING EXERCISES
Rowing 3 to improve scapular stability, shoulder flexibility, and posture	**Thigh Stretch** to speed up recovery of tired legs
Rowing 4 to improve scapular stability, shoulder flexibility, and posture	**Stretch with Pole: Side Down Side Up** to increase flexibility in the torso and hip joint
Pull Straps 2 to improve scapular stability and strengthen rotator cuff muscles	**Stretch with Pole: Front/Back** to improve shoulder flexibility
Teaser One Leg to strengthen torso for serve and stroke	**Stretch Leg Crossed Behind** to speed up recovery of legs and increase hip flexibility
Push-up (advanced) to enhance stamina and dynamic strength	**Calf Stretch** to prevent ankle injury and improve balance
Arm Weights:	
Biceps Curl Front to prevent shoulder injury	
The Bug to improve scapular stability	
Zip Up (on releve) to improve scapular stability	
Shaving (on releve) to improve scapular stability	

STRENGTHENING EXERCISES (continued)	
Lunges to enhance dynamic balance and muscular endurance	
Jump Up to increase lower-body power	
Knee to Chest to enhance dynamic balance, speed	
Wall: Squat One Leg to prevent knee injury and muscular imbalance and endurance	
Arms:	
Wrist Pronation/Supination to prevent wrist injury	
Wrist Raises to prevent wrist injury	
Wrist Rolls to prevent wrist injury	
Ball Squeeze to enhance grip control	

Injury Prevention with Pilates

Tennis stresses most of the areas of the body and nearly all joints are affected by the demands of this game. Injuries generally occur to the shoulder, back, knees, and elbow. Tennis players can use Pilates exercises for strength and stretch as well as proper posture for the foundation of an injury prevention program.

Injuries in tennis players are typically overuse injuries. For example, "tennis elbow" is an overuse injury resulting from repetitive stresses to the outer elbow (tendons that control the wrist and forearm movement). Tennis also places a great deal of stress on the knee joints from bending and quick starts and stops, resulting in overuse injuries like patellar tendinitis (irritation is caused by a lack of support from the surrounding muscles).

SHOULDER

Because of the large range of motion required during play, the shoulder can easily be injured during a tennis match. Therefore muscle imbalance makes the tennis player vulnerable to an overuse injury.

STRENGTHENING	STRETCHING
To stabilize scapular muscles:	To increase range of motion:
Rowing 3 (p. 170)	Roll Up (p. 26)
Rowing 4 (p. 172)	Double Leg Kick (p. 58)
Pull Straps 2 (p. 176)	Wall: Rolling Down (p. 130)
Push-up (p. 122)	Boomerang (p. 96)
Arm Weights: The Bug (p. 152)	Stretch with Pole: Front/Back (p. 198)
Arm Weights: Zip Up (p. 148)	
Arm Weights: Shaving (p. 150)	

Torso and Hips

Training the torso muscles will be beneficial to your best stroke and, combined with strength and flexibility exercises, will help to prevent injury. For strength exercises we stress the sides because the oblique muscles are responsible for torso rotation, which is prevalent in every tennis stroke. Adequate flexibility for the torso and hips is important in preventing lower back injury. Hip flexor and hamstring tightness decreases motion in your hips and stresses your back and can cause lordosis.

TORSO AND HIPS

STRENGTH	STRETCHING
Criss Cross (p. 42)	Roll Up (p. 26)
Corkscrew (p. 48)	Single Leg Circles (p. 30)
Teaser One Leg (p. 178)	Single Leg Stretch (p. 34)
Twist 2 (p. 114)	Single Straight Leg (p. 38)
	Spine Stretch Forward (p. 44)
	Saw (p. 50)
	Spine Twist (p. 64)
	Stretch with Pole: Side Down Side Up (p. 200)
	Stretch Leg Crossed Behind (p. 202)

Lower Back and Abdomen

The lower back and abdominal muscles are an important link between the lower body and upper body as you transfer force from the ground all the way up to the racket.

LOWER BACK AND ABDOMEN

STRENGTH	EXTENSION	STRETCHING
The Hundred (p. 24)	To stabilize the lumbar spine and generate control:	To relieve lower back stress:
Roll Up (p. 26)		Rolling Like a Ball (p. 32)
Roll Over (p. 28)	Swimming (p. 101)	Single Leg Stretch (p. 34)
Single Leg Stretch (p. 34)	Shoulder Bridge (p. 70)	Spine Stretch Forward (p. 44)
Double Leg Stretch (p. 36)	Leg Pull Down (p. 102)	Saw (p. 50)
Single Straight Leg (p. 38)		Seal (p. 124)
Double Straight Leg (p. 40)		Stretch with Pole: Side Down Side Up (p. 200)
Neck Pull (p. 60)		Spine Release Position (p. 285)
Teaser 1 (p. 90)		
Boomerang (p. 96)		

Knee

Quick and sudden pivots cause many knee injuries. It is vital to strengthen the muscles surrounding the knee (especially the quadriceps) in order to stay injury-free. The Pilates exercises below will help to prevent injury from muscular imbalance. When performing knee exercises, always observe knee position to avoid too much pressure between the kneecap and the end of the femur by keeping the leg at a right angle with the thigh and not further forward. Do not hyperextend your knees. If you have a knee injury, make sure to limit your range of motion to decrease stress on the knee. Avoid deep squats and lunges.

Knee

Strengthening	Stretching	Aiding Rehabilitation
Lunge (p. 188)	Roll Up (p. 26)	Standing Leg Flexion (p. 138)
Jump Up (p. 190)	Single Leg Stretch (p. 34)	Seated Leg Extension (p. 136)
Wall: Squat (p. 132)	Single Straight Leg (p. 38)	
Wall: Squat One Leg (p. 134)	Spine Stretch Forward (p. 44)	
	Saw (p. 50)	
	Shoulder Stand Scissors (p. 66)	
	Side Kick: Front/Back (p. 72)	
	Single Leg Kick (p. 56)	
	Thigh Stretch (p. 180)	
	Stretch Leg Crossed Behind (p. 202)	
	Calf Stretch (p. 203)	

Ankle

Ankle sprains are common in tennis because of the quick starts and stops. Strength exercises and flexibility exercises for the calves are necessary for maintaining a healthy ankle. In addition to the exercises below, to strengthen the ankle and practice balance, do the Arm Weights Series (pp. 144–64) on releve, as well as the Towel Exercise (p. 290).

Ankle

Stretching
To improve flexibility:
Leg Pull Down (p. 102)
Calf Stretch (p. 203)
Tennis Ball Exercise (p. 290)

Forearm, Wrists, and Elbow

Tennis elbow (inflamation of the tendon of the forearm extensor muscles) is a common overuse injury for tennis players due to repetitive stress to the forearm muscles. It can also occur from a lack of strength and flexibility in the shoulder. The wrist also receives a great deal of stress from the energy transfered from impact with the ball. The following exercises will work the entire arm.

FOREARM, WRISTS, AND ELBOW

STRENGTHENING	STRETCHING
Arm Weights: Biceps Curls Front (p. 144) Arm Weights: Wrist Raise (p. 158) Arm Weights: Wrist Supination/Pronation (p. 160) Arm Weights: Wrist Rolls (p. 162) Arm Weights: Ball Squeeze (p. 164) Castanets (p. 292)	Forearm Flexor Stretch: With the elbow straight and the forearm supinated (palm up), use the opposite hand to stretch the wrist back. Forearm Extensor Stretch: With the elbow straight and the forearm pronated (palm down), use the opposite hand to stretch the wrist downward.

Tennis Routines

In the off-season, practice each of the tennis programs twice per week.
During the season, practice each workout once per week.

WORKOUT 1

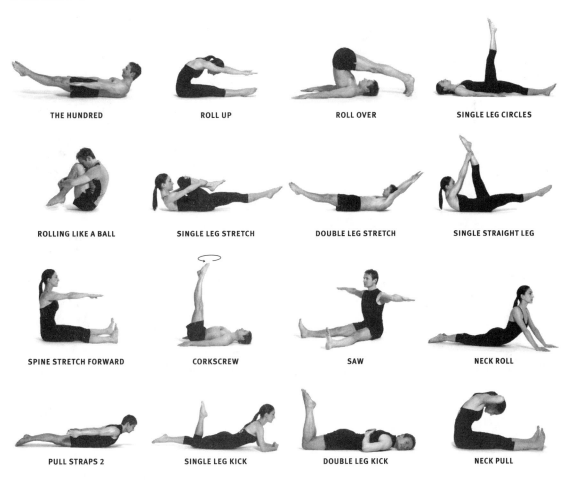

THE HUNDRED

ROLL UP

ROLL OVER

SINGLE LEG CIRCLES

ROLLING LIKE A BALL

SINGLE LEG STRETCH

DOUBLE LEG STRETCH

SINGLE STRAIGHT LEG

SPINE STRETCH FORWARD

CORKSCREW

SAW

NECK ROLL

PULL STRAPS 2

SINGLE LEG KICK

DOUBLE LEG KICK

NECK PULL

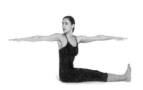

SPINE TWIST

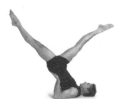

SHOULDER STAND SCISSORS

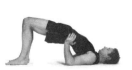

SHOULDER BRIDGE

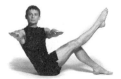

TEASER ONE LEG

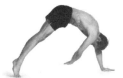

TWIST 2

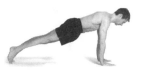

PUSH-UP

SEAL

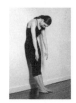

WALL: ROLLING DOWN

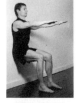

WALL: SQUAT

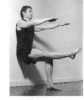

WALL: SQUAT ONE LEG

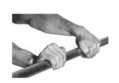

ARM WEIGHTS: WRIST ROLLS

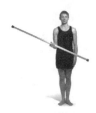

**ARM WEIGHTS:
SUPINATION/PRONATION**

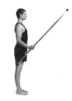

ARM WEIGHTS: WRIST RAISE

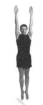

JUMP UP

STRETCH LEG CROSSED BEHIND

WORKOUT 2

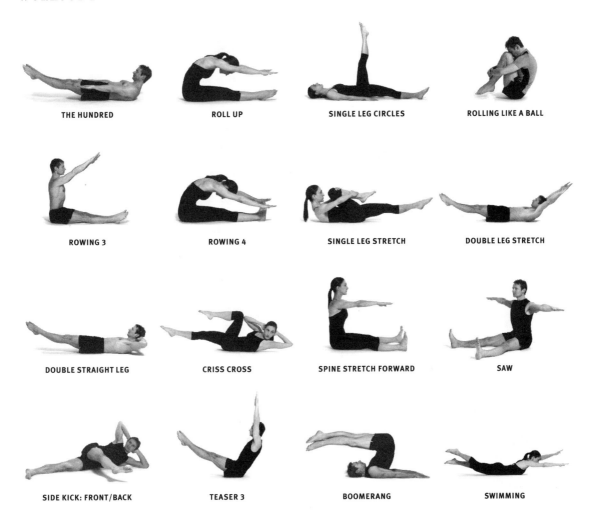

THE HUNDRED   ROLL UP   SINGLE LEG CIRCLES   ROLLING LIKE A BALL

ROWING 3   ROWING 4   SINGLE LEG STRETCH   DOUBLE LEG STRETCH

DOUBLE STRAIGHT LEG   CRISS CROSS   SPINE STRETCH FORWARD   SAW

SIDE KICK: FRONT/BACK   TEASER 3   BOOMERANG   SWIMMING

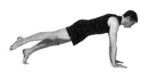

LEG PULL DOWN

THIGH STRETCH

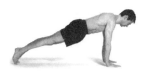

PUSH-UP

SEAL

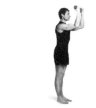

ARM WEIGHTS: BICEPS CURL FRONT

ARM WEIGHTS: THE BUG

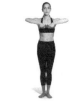

ARM WEIGHTS: ZIP UP

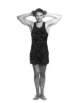

ARM WEIGHTS: SHAVING

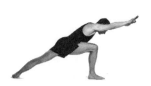

LUNGES

KNEE TO CHEST

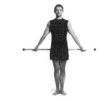

STRETCH WITH POLE: FRONT/BACK

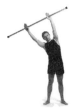

STRETCH WITH POLE: SIDE DOWN SIDE UP

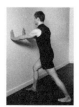

CALF STRETCH

15

Pilates Solutions to Common Sports-Related Aches and Pains

Joseph Pilates was considered one of the first physiotherapists.

Dancers were among the first professional athletes to turn to Pilates for

fitness and injury prevention. Today, doctors and physical therapists

alike are familiar with the Pilates method and are supportive of its

benefits because Pilates helps to achieve healing through movement.

By correcting muscle imbalance and correctly strengthening muscles, Pilates can help people suffering from back, shoulder, knee, and hip pain, as well as sciatica, headaches, and stiff and weak necks. The mini-programs found in this chapter have been designed especially for the needs of the various sports cited in this book. The exercises should be used as long as necessary, either to rehabilitate injuries or to improve weaknesses.

However, Pilates is a not a quick fix and ideally should be used on a daily basis as a maintenance program. Pilates is an effective therapy for sports injuries such as treating torn ligaments. Once the break or strain has begun to heal, practicing Pilates will help to speed the healing process by stretching and remobilizing injured muscles and stiffened joints.

Athletes often continue to train despite the fact that they feel pain. Pain should be treated as a warning signal from your body. It is essential to be able to discern between the pain of muscle soreness and true injury. During hard training, in anaerobic activity, when there is insufficient oxygen from the blood to maintain aerobic metabolism, a by-product of anaerobic glycolysis is lactic acid. Lactic acid accumulates in the muscle and is responsible for the burning sensation you may feel when you exercise. This soreness is acceptable pain, and by training and maintaining a good diet, the body improves at quickly removing the lactic acid. Injuries, on the other hand, are torn muscles and ligaments, as well as stress injuries, which can impair your overall fitness level.

One of the main causes of injury for athletes is the overuse of one side of the body. In activities like golf and tennis, one-sided movements lead to injury by overdeveloping one side and create an imbalance between your strong side and your weak side. Pilates balances the body by working evenly, developing better body symmetry, and thereby correcting muscle imbalance. In addition, we have added extra repetitions for the weaker side and extra stretches for the tighter side in the routines.

Lack of strength and flexibility can also contribute to injury. In any particular sport, an athlete focuses on a specific movement, using only certain muscles and neglecting others, which could cause injury. Pilates strengthens the whole body, developing small muscle groups as well as large muscle groups. Using Pilates, cyclists improve their cycling stroke not only by working their quadriceps, but also by strengthening the powerhouse because when their movement initiates from the center, they can perform with greater strength and efficiency. Flexibility is important in all sports, such as the tennis serve, the back swing in golf, and for the position of your back in cycling. Lack of flexibility increases the chance of pulling or tearing muscles. Pilates increases your flexibility because each exercise combines both stretch and strength components.

Working outside the frame of the body often puts undue stress on the joints. In tennis, when you swing at a ball that is out of reach you can pull your back by overextension. The Pilates routine stresses the importance of working within the frame of the body ("in the box") to better prepare the body to handle the strains inherent in these physical activities.

When you are unaware of your body's movement you can injure yourself by lack of movement control. Pilates teaches body awareness by keeping your mind focused on the task at hand. When you are doing Pilates you focus on controlling your movements and this continued attention will develop your awareness of how the body moves, which will ultimately enhance your athletic performance.

The two most common sports injury categories are muscle injuries and tendon injuries. When muscles are overused or put to use without first being warmed up, they can either tear or go into spasms. It is common for athletes to permanently abandon their sport because of their injuries. Pilates is an effective method for repairing injuries and will help to regenerate body tissue. Because it is a workout designed to uniformly develop the body, Pilates is an excellent method of strengthening weak joints and muscles, stretching tight tendons and muscles, and correcting muscular imbalance around the joints. When performing Pilates exercises, you will drive pure, fresh blood to every muscle of your body. The blood flows through the muscles to supply them with sufficient oxygen and nutrients to do their job and also eliminate the waste products created by fatigue, and will help muscles heal quickly.

After becoming injured, you should first allow the injury to heal as quickly as possible (whether it be applying heat, ice, or taking medical advice from your doctor). Refrain from doing anything that would stress the injury until the swelling or pain has subsided. Finally, begin to rebuild strength and flexibility in the injured area as soon as possible in order to prevent muscle atrophy.

The following is a quick reference guide to common injuries and body issues that are a result of fatigue and overuse in training. The exercises listed are all part of the Pilates system and should be done with respect to the whole method. Learn the exercises as part of the entire routine, and you may then use them individually as you feel necessary. If you experience pain while exercising, stop the exercise and return to it when you feel stronger.

Back Pain

Back pain is frequently the result of tight hip flexors. When biking, running, playing golf, tennis, skiing, and swimming, the hip and thigh muscles shorten and the back muscles can spasm. The goal is to relax them and to strengthen the powerhouse, correct postural problems such as lordosis, and stretch the lower back, hamstrings, and hip flexor muscles.

The following exercises can be done for minor back pain. If you are experiencing serious back pain such as spondylolisthesis (displacement of the fifth lumbar vertebra) or a herniated disk (unusual pressure between two adjacent vertebrae with the intervertebral disk sticking out), you should consult with a physician before starting any kind of exercise.

- The Hundred—modified (p. 24)

- Roll Up—modified (p. 26)

- Single Leg Circles—modified (p. 30)

- Single Leg Stretch—modified (p. 34)

- Double Leg Stretch—modified (p. 36)

- Spine Stretch Forward (p. 44)

- Swimming—modified (p. 101): keep the back (lumbar spine) supported by the abdominal muscles and lengthen your limbs out. First extend your arms and pump them up and down, breathing in for five counts, then out for five counts. Repeat 2 sets. Then keeping the arms extended but still, reach your legs out and start kicking legs, breathing in the same manner as above. Repeat 2 sets.

- Spine Stretch Release: Lying on your stomach, place your palms on the mat at chest level with your elbows pointed upward. Push against the mat with your hands and bend your knees, lifting your upper body off the floor and backward until you are sitting on your heels. Keep your upper body bent over your knees, but your stomach lifted off your thighs. Your arms should be extended straight from the shoulders with palms still in their original position on the mat. Your head and neck should be relaxed.

- Spine Release Position: Lie on your back and bring your knees into your body in the fetal position. Wrap your arms around your legs, hugging them as you bring them close into the chest. Keep a long neck and torso, with your stomach and ribs pulled in.

- Wall: Arm Circles (p. 128)

- Wall: Rolling Down (p. 130)

- Wall: Squat (p. 132)

Sciatica, which can be caused by poor posture, a weak powerhouse, or twisted hips, is a pain that radiates down from the buttocks, occasionally down the leg, and all the way to the foot. For pain on both sides perform the following exercises:

- Spine Stretch Release (see above)

- Pelvic Curl (Shoulder Bridge, modified) (p. 70): Lie on your back with knees bent and feet flat on the floor. Pull the hip-bones to the rib cage so that your pelvis tilts off the floor. Try not to use your feet to push up and do not arch your back.

For one-sided sciatica, avoid contracting the lower back muscles on the side where the pain is located, in order to avoid pressing on the sciatic nerve. The tight side of the back should be stretched. Do the following exercises, adding an extra stretch to the tight side (*):

- The Hundred—modified (p. 24)

- Single Leg Stretch (p. 34)

- Double Leg Stretch—modified (p. 36)

- Side Kick: Bicycle (p. 78)

- Side Kick: Double Leg Lift—modified (p. 80)

- Spine Twist (p. 64)

- Swimming—modified (p. 101)

- Stretch with Pole: Side Down Side Up—modified (p. 200)

For lumbar lordosis, which is an increased pelvic inclination (an arched lower back that pushes the pelvis forward) and tight hip flexors, practice the following:

- The Hundred—modified (p. 24)

- Roll Up—modified (p. 26)

- Single Leg Circles (p. 30)

- Single Leg Stretch (p. 34)

- Double Leg Stretch—modified (p. 36)

- Spine Stretch Forward (p. 44)

- Shoulder Bridge—modified (p. 70)

- Wall: Arm Circles (p. 128)

- Wall: Rolling Down (p. 130)

- Spine Release Position (p. 283)

- Spine Stretch Release (p. 285)

Scoliosis is both lateral flexion and rotation of the spine, which results in both tight and weak muscles. To check for scoliosis, test the strength and mobility on both sides. If a strength exercise, such as Side Kick: Double Leg Lift (p. 80) or Arm Weights: The Bug (p. 152), is more difficult on one side, do 3 to 5 extra repetitions on that side. If a stretch exercise, such as Arm Weights: Side to Side (p. 146), is more difficult on one side, hold the stretch longer on that side.

- The Hundred—modified (p. 24)

- Roll Up (p. 26)

- Single Leg Stretch (p. 34)

- Double Leg Stretch—modified (p. 36)

- Side Kick: Double Leg Lift (p. 80)

- Swimming (p. 101) (if powerhouse is strong enough)

- Mermaid—modified: keep the focus on the tighter side and hold the stretch position longer (p. 108)

- Twist 1 (p.112) (if strong enough)

- Stretch with Pole: Side Down Side Up—modified (p. 200)

- Arm Weights: Side to Side: focus on the tighter side and hold the stretch position longer on that side (p. 146)

Neck and Shoulder Tension

If you experience strain in your neck as a result of hard training, because of nervous tension before a race, or due to bad habits working at the office, the result is that you contract your neck and upper back (trapezius and levator scapulae) muscles. This muscular tension produces poor posture and a negative effect on the execution of many activities, such as the tennis serve or the back swing in golf, by reducing the range of motion of shoulder flexion when lifting your arm above your head. It is therefore important to stretch the neck muscles. When doing neck exercises, hold the stretch position, inhale a deep breath, and exhale when you come back to center.

- Shoulder Rolls: roll shoulders forward in a circle 5 times, then reverse.

- Shoulder Elevation: Inhale, lift your shoulders to your ears, and hold. Then drop and exhale. Repeat 5 times.

- Neck Turns: In a seated position, turn your head to the right side, then look to the left side. Repeat 2 times on each side.

- Neck to Side: In a seated position, looking straight ahead, bend your neck and reach your ear to your shoulder. Come back to center and switch to the other side. Repeat 2 times on each side.

- Neck Circles: In a seated position, tilt your head to one side, then roll down and around to the other side and up. *Do not* roll your head back as it crunches the neck. Repeat once in each direction.

- Neck Roll (p. 52)

- Snake (p. 110)

- Wall: Rolling Down (with weights) (p. 130)—this exercise will aid circulation around the shoulder joint and vertebrae.

- Stretch with Pole: Front/Back (p. 198)

To strengthen the neck muscles and correct bad posture:

- Wall: Neck Exercise—modified (p. 140)

- Neck Extension: Lie on the floor with a shallow cushion under your head. Push the back of your head into the cushion and hold it for 10 counts. Relax for 10 counts. Repeat three times.

To strengthen the shoulders:

- Arm Weights: Zip Up (p. 148)

- Arm Weights: Shaving (p. 150)

- Arm Weights: The Bug (p. 152)

Tired Legs

Speed up the process of recovery, increase flexibility, and facilitate elimination of the products of fatigue with the following:

- Saw (p. 50)

- Side Kick: Front/Back (p. 72)

- Side Kick: Bicycle (p. 78)

- Shoulder Stand Scissors (p. 66)

- Shoulder Stand Bicycle (p. 68)

- Balance Control (p. 120)

- Seal (p. 124)

- Calf Stretch (p. 203)

- Stretch Leg Crossed Behind (p. 202)

To facilitate blood flow in the feet and legs and strengthen the feet:

- Towel Exercise: Sit on a chair with a towel laid lengthwise on the floor under your bare feet, keeping your heels on the end of the towel closest to you. Alternate one foot at a time, gripping the toes to bunch the towel up under you. The towel should bunch up under your feet. Then reverse, pushing the towel away, or un-bunching it.

- Tennis Ball Exercise: Sitting on a chair or standing, place a tennis ball under one foot. Massage the foot by rolling the ball back and forth.

Knee Pain

Due to the complexity of the joint and abnormal positioning (such as knocked knees or bowed legs), the knee is frequently injured in many sports. In most cases, incorrect tracking of the patella causes pain in the front of the knee over the knee. In the runner and biker, misalignment of the foot and knee are causes of the problem. For the tennis player and skier, knee injuries are caused by quick pivots and landing incorrectly from a jump. The swimmer puts stress on the knee during the breaststroke. For injury rehabilitation, correcting the posture and aligning the hip, knee, and foot reduces pressure on the joints.

When you have knee pain, keep the knees soft—do not lock or hyperextend your knees. It is necessary to strengthen the knee flexors and extensors and lateral and medial stabilizers to add stability to the knee joint.

- Side Kick: Front/Back (p. 72)

- Side Kick: Bicycle (p. 78)

- Footwork 1 (p. 166)

- Footwork 2 (p. 168)

- Standing Leg Flexion (p. 138)

- Seated Leg Extension—modified (p. 136)

Tight Hamstrings and Hip Flexors

Hamstring muscles may be more susceptible to injury due to high forces and excessive stress during movements with excessive hip flexion, as in the gait cycle while running. Tight hamstrings restrict flexibility for runners and limit the range of motion in the gait cycle. They can also be a cause of lordosis.

- Roll Up (p. 26)

- Roll Over (p. 28)

- Single Leg Circles (p. 30)

- Single Leg Stretch (p. 34)

- Single Straight Leg (p. 38)

- Spine Stretch Forward (p. 44)

- Saw (p. 50)

- Shoulder Stand Scissors (p. 66)

- Shoulder Stand Bicycle (p. 68)

- Side Kicks—the entire series (pp. 72–88)

- Rocking (p. 116)

- Calf Stretch (p. 203)

Elbows and Wrists

In tennis and golf, the elbow joint is susceptible to overuse injury. Repetitive bending and rotating movements of the forearm increase tension in the wrist and elbow muscles and cause tennis elbow. In cycling one puts excess pressure on the wrists when controlling the bike downhill, while the skier puts pressure on the wrists during pole planting.

- Arm Weights: Low Curls (p. 156)

- Arm Weights: Ball Squeeze (p. 164)

- Arm Weights: Wrist Rolls (p. 162)

- Arm Weights: Wrist Raises (p. 158)

- Arm Weights: Wrist: Supination/Pronation (p. 160)

- Castanets: In a standing position, raise your arms shoulder height, palms facing each other. Slightly bend the elbows to the sides. Tap each finger to your thumb 10 times consecutively, then reverse. Repeat 1 time each direction.

Appendix: Complete Mat Program

The following pages illustrate the complete mat program, in the order in which it should be done. We have broken it down into three separate routines—beginner, intermediate, and advanced—so that you can see how the entire program progresses and how the exercises flow from one to the next.

The Beginner Mat Program

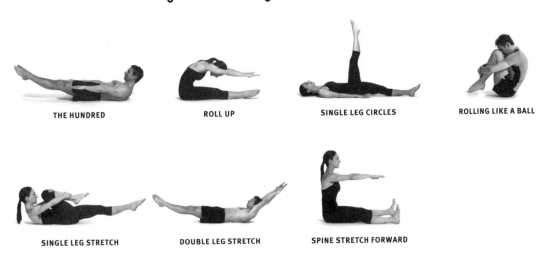

THE HUNDRED

ROLL UP

SINGLE LEG CIRCLES

ROLLING LIKE A BALL

SINGLE LEG STRETCH

DOUBLE LEG STRETCH

SPINE STRETCH FORWARD

The Intermediate Mat Program

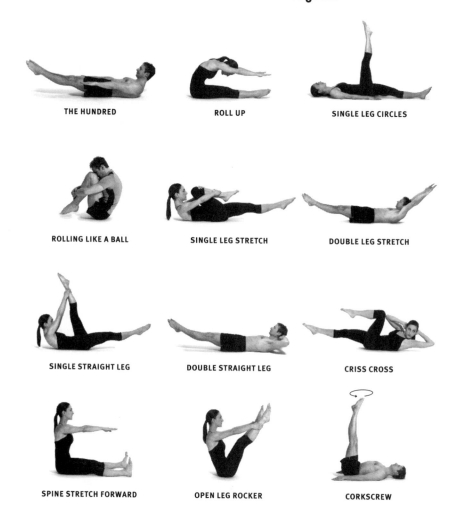

THE HUNDRED

ROLL UP

SINGLE LEG CIRCLES

ROLLING LIKE A BALL

SINGLE LEG STRETCH

DOUBLE LEG STRETCH

SINGLE STRAIGHT LEG

DOUBLE STRAIGHT LEG

CRISS CROSS

SPINE STRETCH FORWARD

OPEN LEG ROCKER

CORKSCREW

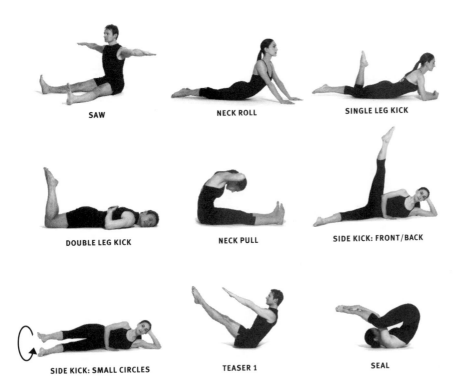

SAW

NECK ROLL

SINGLE LEG KICK

DOUBLE LEG KICK

NECK PULL

SIDE KICK: FRONT/BACK

SIDE KICK: SMALL CIRCLES

TEASER 1

SEAL

The Advanced Mat Program

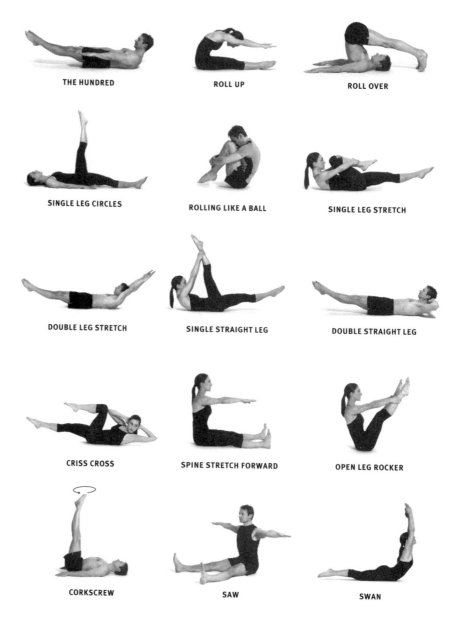

THE HUNDRED

ROLL UP

ROLL OVER

SINGLE LEG CIRCLES

ROLLING LIKE A BALL

SINGLE LEG STRETCH

DOUBLE LEG STRETCH

SINGLE STRAIGHT LEG

DOUBLE STRAIGHT LEG

CRISS CROSS

SPINE STRETCH FORWARD

OPEN LEG ROCKER

CORKSCREW

SAW

SWAN

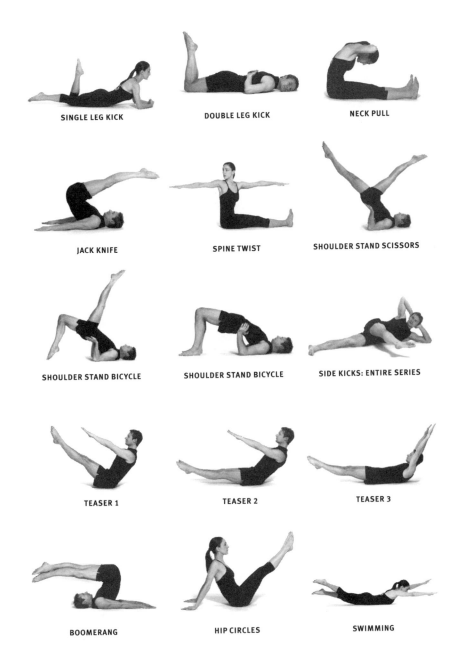

SINGLE LEG KICK

DOUBLE LEG KICK

NECK PULL

JACK KNIFE

SPINE TWIST

SHOULDER STAND SCISSORS

SHOULDER STAND BICYCLE

SHOULDER STAND BICYCLE

SIDE KICKS: ENTIRE SERIES

TEASER 1

TEASER 2

TEASER 3

BOOMERANG

HIP CIRCLES

SWIMMING

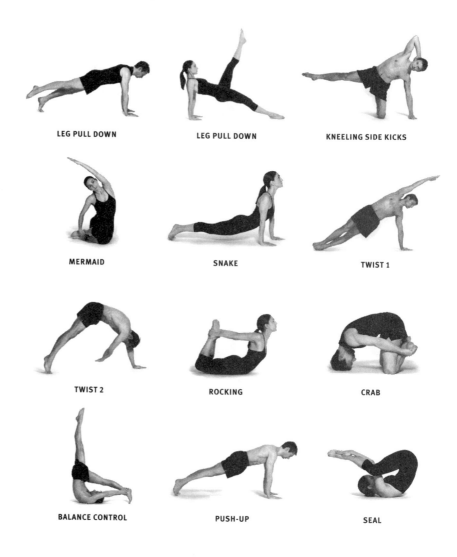

LEG PULL DOWN

LEG PULL DOWN

KNEELING SIDE KICKS

MERMAID

SNAKE

TWIST 1

TWIST 2

ROCKING

CRAB

BALANCE CONTROL

PUSH-UP

SEAL

Glossary

abduction. Movement of a joint in the frontal plane, so that the limb moves away from the center of the body.

adduction. Movement of a joint in the frontal plane, so that the limb moves toward the center of the body.

aerobic metabolism. Metabolism in the cell that takes place in the presence of oxygen.

anaerobic metabolism. Metabolism in the cell that takes place when there is not sufficient oxygen supplied by the blood to maintain aerobic metabolism.

ankle dorso flexor and plantar flexor. Muscles responsible for the flexion and extension of the ankle.

atrophy. Loss of muscle tone, size, and strength.

biceps. The elbow flexor muscles found at the front of the upper arm.

cartilage. Connective tissue that is found at the end of a bone.

cervical spine. The seven vertebrae of the neck.

deltoid muscles. Anterior, middle, and posterior deltoids combine to form a cap sleeve of the muscle over the top of the shoulder joint.

endorphins. Hormones released in the body in response to stress to reduce the sensation of pain.

erector spinae muscles. Extensor muscles of the spine that run along the spine from the neck to the lumbar spine.

extension. Movement of a joint in the sagittal plane; the act of straightening a limb.

fascia. Matter that separates muscles from adjacent muscles.

flexion. Movement of a joint in the sagittal plane; the act of bending a limb.

gastrocnemius. The calf muscles.

glenohumeral. The shoulder joint that is between the head of the humerus and the glenoid fossa (socket) of the scapula.

gluteal muscles. Gluteus maximus, medius, and minimus, the posterior muscles of the hip joint.

glycolysis. Breakdown of carbohydrates as glucose and glycogen by enzymes with the release of energy and production of lactic acid.

hamstrings. The three muscles of the back of the legs.

hip adductor/abductor muscles. Function as adduction and abduction of hip joint.

hip extensor/flexor muscles. Function as extension and flexion of the hip joint.

hypertrophy. Increase in size and strength of a muscle.

hypomobility. Loss of range of motion of a joint.

hypovascularity. Decrease in blood flow.

IT band (ilio-tibial band). The ligament that runs along the outside of the thigh from the top of the hip to the knee.

kyphosis. Abnormal convex curvature of the spine.

lactic acid. A by-product of anaerobic metabolism that cannot be used effectively by working muscles.

lateral and medial stabilizers. The abductor and adductor muscles that stabilize the knee and hip joints.

latisimus dorsi. The largest muscle of the back that is responsible for shoulder internal rotation, adduction, and extension.

levator scapulae. The muscles responsible for scapular elevation and stabilization.

ligaments. Connective tissue that attaches bone to bone.

lordosis. Abnormal forward curvature of the spine resulting in a sway-backed posture.

lumbar spine. The five vertebrae of the lower back.

lumbopelvic area. The area where articulation of the sacrum and hip bones occurs.

obliques (external/internal). Waistline muscles that rotate the torso.

para spinal muscles. A group of muscles running along the spine.

pectoralis major. Big chest muscle attaches all along the breastbone and collarbone to the bicipital groove of the humerus.

pectoralis minor. Muscle that pulls the shoulder downward.

pronation. Movement of a joint toward the prone position (toward the floor).

psoas iliaque. The most powerful hip muscle that is responsible for hip flexion, adduction, and external rotation and that flexes the trunk toward the leg.

quadriceps. The muscles of the front of the thigh that act as the knee extensor and assist in flexing the hip joint (rectus femoris).

rectus femoris. The front of the thigh, the major quadriceps muscle.

rhomboids. The muscles responsible for fixation of the scapula.

rotary flexibility. The rotation that is a motion around a central axis.

rotator cuff. Group of dynamic stabilizers of the glenohumeral joint responsible for maintaining congruency of the humeral head in the glenoid fossa.

scapula. The shoulder blade, a bone forming the back part of the shoulder.

sciatica. Pain involving the sciatic nerve, often felt in the lower back and along the back of the thigh.

shoulder complex. Articulation between the humerus and the glenoid fossa of the scapula (glenohumeral joint) and the scapula with the thorax (scapulothoracic joint).

subscapularis. A rotator cuff muscle that stabilizes the humeral head in the glenoid cavity during shoulder movement.

supination. Movement of a joint toward the supine position (toward the ceiling).

tendinitis. Inflammation of the tendon, which could take place in the ankle, shoulder, elbow, etc.

tendons. Connective tissue that attaches muscle to bone.

teres major. Shoulder muscles that allow scapular movement such as shoulder internal rotation, adduction, and extension.

teres minor. A rotator cuff muscle that rotates the shoulder externally.

thoracic spine. Part of the spine between the neck and abdomen, composed of twelve vertebrae.

trapezius. The large muscle divided into three major sections: upper, middle, and lower trapezius—that elevate, adduct, upward rotate, and depress the scapula.

triceps. The elbow extensor muscles found at the back of the upper arm.

Index

Note: *Italic* numbers indicate illustrations.

About the Authors

Karrie Adamany and Daniel Loigerot graduated from the Pilates Certification Program in New York City under the tutelage of Romana Kryzanowska, master teacher, who was personally chosen by Joseph Pilates to carry on his teaching. In order to ensure the highest quality of teaching to their own students, they continue to work closely with Kryzanowska and to teach at her training center.

Adamany and Loigerot own the Pilates Edge Studio in SoHo in New York City. In their customized private space they offer Pilates lessons tailored to their clients' individualized needs. Their personal approach has won them a loyal following.

Karrie Adamany is the founder of ab lab®, a service that sends certified Pilates instructors to hotels and private residences. She has been featured in various publications such as *Elle*, *Gotham*, *Australian Vogue*, and *In New York*. She studied Pilates intensely for several years before becoming a certified instructor. A graduate of the University of Minnesota, she is also a writer and a mother. Adamany is currently developing a Pilates program designed specifically for women recuperating from childbirth.

Daniel Loigerot opened his first training center in Marseille in 1987. He organized and instructed private classes for professional athletes, including triathletes, marathon runners, soccer, basketball and tennis players, cyclists, and golfers. He was also a personal trainer for both the French National II Basketball Team and the French National II Cycling Team. As a trainer, he designed comprehensive health and fitness evaluations incorporating components of strength, flexibility, and cardiovascular and muscular endurance. He is a former French National triathlete, competing three times in the world championships from 1990 to 1996.

Loigerot is a graduate of the Sport University, Marseille, France, in sciences and techniques of physical education and sports (Department of Athletic Training). He also holds degrees in sports and health and general studies, with a specialization in the sciences, from the University of Aix-Marseille II, as well as a degree in cellular biology from the Science University in Marseille. He is a certified personal trainer and martial arts instructor in judo.